Reversing the Obesogenic Environment

Physical Activity Intervention Series

Rebecca E. Lee, PhD
University of Houston

Kristen M. McAlexander, PhD
Southern Methodist University

Jorge A. Banda, MS
University of South Carolina

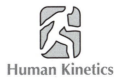

Human Kinetics

Library of Congress Cataloging-in-Publication Data

Lee, Rebecca E., 1966-
  Reversing the obesogenic environment / Rebecca E. Lee, Kristen McAlexander, Jorge Banda.
    p. cm. -- (Physical activity intervention series)
  Includes bibliographical references and index.
  ISBN-13: 978-0-7360-7899-3 (softcover)
  ISBN-10: 0-7360-7899-1 (softcover)
  1. Obesity--Epidemiology. 2. Obesity--Exercise therapy. 3. Obesity--Prevention. I. McAlexander,
Kristen, 1981- II. Banda, Jorge, 1978- III. Title.
  RC628.L37 2011
  362.196'398--dc22

                                    2010043031

ISBN-10: 0-7360-7899-1 (print)
ISBN-13: 978-0-7360-7899-3 (print)

Copyright © 2011 by Rebecca E. Lee, Kristen M. McAlexander, and Jorge A. Banda

The Web addresses cited in this text were current as of October 2010, unless otherwise noted.

Acquisitions Editor: Myles Schrag; **Developmental Editor:** Amanda S. Ewing; **Assistant Editors:** Antoinette Pomata and Steven Calderwood; **Copyeditor:** Mary Rivers; **Indexer:** Susan Danzi Hernandez; **Permission Manager:** Martha Gullo; **Graphic Designer:** Joe Buck; **Graphic Artists:** Nancy Rasmus and Kathleen Boudreau-Fuoss; **Cover Designer:** Keith Blomberg; **Photographer (cover):** © Human Kinetics; **Photographer (interior):** © Human Kinetics unless otherwise noted. Photo on page 15 © Roy Morsch/age fotostock; photo on page 47 © Wilmar/age fotostock; photo on page 75 © Sonderegger Christof/Prisma/age fotostock; photo on page 89 © Kristian Cabanis/age fotostock; photo on page 105 © Jim West/age fotostock; photo on page 121 © Dennis MacDonald/age fotostock; photo on page 149 © Ariel Skelley/age fotostock; photo on page 179 © John Birdsall/CMSP; **Photo Asset Manager:** Laura Fitch; **Art Manager:** Kelly Hendren; **Associate Art Manager:** Alan L. Wilborn; **Illustrations:** © Human Kinetics; **Printer:** Sheridan Books

Printed in the United States of America   10   9   8   7   6   5   4   3   2   1

The paper in this book is certified under a sustainable forestry program.

Human Kinetics
Web site: www.HumanKinetics.com

United States: Human Kinetics
P.O. Box 5076
Champaign, IL 61825-5076
800-747-4457
e-mail: humank@hkusa.com

Canada: Human Kinetics
475 Devonshire Road Unit 100
Windsor, ON N8Y 2L5
800-465-7301 (in Canada only)
e-mail: info@hkcanada.com

Europe: Human Kinetics
107 Bradford Road
Stanningley
Leeds LS28 6AT, United Kingdom
+44 (0) 113 255 5665
e-mail: hk@hkeurope.com

Australia: Human Kinetics
57A Price Avenue
Lower Mitcham, South Australia 5062
08 8372 0999
e-mail: info@hkaustralia.com

New Zealand: Human Kinetics
P.O. Box 80
Torrens Park, South Australia 5062
0800 222 062
e-mail: info@hknewzealand.com

E4674

CONTENTS

PART I   Public Health and Obesity   1

CHAPTER 1   Emergence of the Obesogenic Environment 3

CHAPTER 2   Scope of Obesity 15

CHAPTER 3   Body Composition Measurements 29

PART II   Physical Activity and Obesity   45

CHAPTER 4   The Built Environment 47

PART V   Media and Marketing   177

SERIES PREFACE

The purpose of the Physical Activity Intervention Series is to publish texts, written by the leading researchers in the field, that provide specific and evidence-based methods and techniques for physical activity interventions. These books include practical suggestions, examples, forms, questionnaires, and intervention techniques that can be applied in field settings.

Many health professionals who currently provide exercise advice and offer exercise programs use the traditional and structured frequency, intensity, and time (FIT) approach to exercise prescription. Although the exercise prescription is valid, going to a fitness facility and participating in such programs are not attractive to many people. Alternative programs based on the new consensus recommendations and using behavioral intervention methods and techniques are needed.

The books in the Physical Activity Intervention Series provide information, methods, techniques, and support to the many health professionals—clinical exercise physiologists, nutritionists, physicians, fitness center exercise leaders, public health workers, and health promotion experts—who are looking for alternative ways to promote physical activity that do not require a rigid application of the FIT approach. It is to meet this need that Human Kinetics developed this Physical Activity Intervention Series.

The series has a broad scope. It includes books focused on after-school programs for children and youth, ways to implement physical activity interventions in the public health setting, and ways to evaluate physical activity interventions. The series also includes books that focus on the implementation of interventions based on theories and on interventions for other special populations such as older adults and those with chronic disease. Each book is valuable and useful in its own right, but the series will provide an integrated collection of materials that can be used to plan, develop, implement, and evaluate physical activity interventions in a wide variety of settings for diverse populations.

PREFACE

Obesity is a crisis. Some scholars call it an epidemic because over one third of the general population is obese and another third is overweight. Other scholars have done statistical projections that show that by the middle of the 21st century, if things continue as they have been for the last 30 years, the entire U.S. population will be obese, soon followed by the world. National leaders worry about national security, terrorist attacks, and other crises as potential threats to global stability, but we really need look no further than home, our kitchens and living rooms, where we grow bigger and bigger. As obesity prevalence continues to rise, so do associated health care costs, employment costs, and transportation costs, as well as many other hidden costs associated with the grand expansion of America.

On average, between the ages of 25 and 55, Americans gain 1 pound, or .5 kilogram, of fat per year, while they lose half a pound of muscle tissue per year. If someone is overweight at age 25, obesity is already a fait accompli. Most people are mere time bombs in a well-documented cascade of health-compromising conditions and medical expenses that lead to a reduced life span and a reduced quality of life for their remaining years. The fundamental cause of obesity is too many calories consumed (dietary habits or overeating) and too few calories expended (physical activity or the lack thereof). Although this seems obvious to scholars and practitioners, the process that leads to this calorie imbalance is slow and insidious.

Recent research has confirmed numerous genetic predisposing factors that lead to obesity; however, the recent explosion in obesity prevalence is not driven primarily by genetic or biological factors. First, although there are many genetic predisposing factors, there is no single gene or genetic combination prototype that is reliably identified in obese individuals. Second, and more important, humans have had the same genetic makeup for thousands of years, so no sudden genetic shift is to blame for the obesity epidemic. What has changed in recent history is our environment. We have the same genes that humans have had for centuries, but now we are faced with an obesogenic environment.

Obesogenic is a term that was coined in the mid-1990s to refer to situations or conditions that lead to people becoming increasingly obese. The word *obesogenic* is a combination of the words *obese* and *genic*—something that creates or leads to obesity. Something in our environments is leading us to become obese. The billion dollar question then is this: "What is it?" Strong evidence first came from the social epidemiologists who found that, in the United States and many other industrialized nations, regardless of who you were—

your education, your income, your marital status, your race—the likelihood you were overweight or obese depended upon where you lived. For example, people who lived in neighborhoods made up of, in general, individuals with lower educational attainment and lower paying jobs were more likely to be overweight or obese compared to people living in neighborhoods of residents with more education and higher paying jobs. The remarkable thing was that it did not matter who the individual was—residents were interchangeable. Regardless of what walk of life they came from, people were more likely to be overweight or obese if they lived in these so-called "deprived" neighborhoods.

The challenge with social epidemiology studies is that the data are based on aggregate data, so it is impossible to determine what the specific, manifest characteristics of the obesogenic neighborhoods were. Was it the lack of fresh fruits and vegetables? Was it the lack of safe places to be physically active? Was it the oppressive lack of neighborhood curb appeal? Perhaps it was something else. Maybe these neighborhoods had more fast food restaurants, greater reliance on automobiles, or greater marketing efforts by snack food companies. Perhaps it was all of these factors and more. Often, concerned communities will attempt to take action, but unless efforts occur at multiple levels in the system, it is difficult to have sustainable results. Sometimes, too, some groups of the population will exhibit particular vulnerabilities to obesity, and the emphasis is shifted to individual factors associated with these individuals, such as sex, race, or ethnicity. It is likely that those individual factors are a very small part of the problem, and much broader efforts are needed.

This book is intended to help recognize the many factors that lead to an obesogenic environment and propose how we, collectively, can work to reverse those factors. To that end, this book is organized into five sections. Although nearly everything in this book is related to other parts of the book, it makes sense conceptually to organize the book into separate chapters that can be read as stand-alone references on a topic, combined with other related chapters in a section, or taken together with the other chapters in the book. Part I, Public Health and Obesity, provides the background and foundation for the remaining chapters in the book. The first chapter, Emergence of the Obesogenic Environment, provides a brief historical perspective and theoretically grounds the book in an ecologic framework. The next chapter, Scope of Obesity, provides information on the prevalence of obesity, discusses particularly vulnerable populations, and illustrates the risks of obesity. The last chapter in this first part of the book, Body Composition Measurements, describes the measurement of obesity, with particular attention paid to methods used in public health and community settings.

The second part of the book, Physical Activity and Obesity, discusses neighborhood and home environmental factors related to physical activity. Chapter 4, The Built Environment, defines and describes components of the built environment that influence physical activity and discusses how these are measured and quantified. We present an overview of the limitations and current understanding of the knowledge base and comment on some emerging directions. Chapter 5, Physical Activity Resources, describes common types of physical activity resources, how they are measured, and their role in the promotion of physical activity and prevention of obesity. Chapter 6, Active Transportation, defines and describes active transportation systems, both outdoor and indoor, and how active transportation is related to physical activity and obesity.

The third part of the book, Food Accessibility, describes how food production and technology directly and indirectly affect obesity. Chapter 7, Food Supply and Security, discusses how the food supply has contributed to the nutrition transition and the resulting nutritional disparities: obesity and undernutrition. This is followed by an overview of food security, the interventions and programs that have been developed in response to this issue, and their impact on obesity. Chapter 8, Food Technology, discusses the trend toward biotechnological innovation and the impact this has on the food supply, dietary habits, obesity, and health.

The fourth section, Public Policy, Sociocultural Influences, and Obesity, highlights social factors such as cultural beliefs and policies that influence obesity. Chapter 9, Policy and Individual Health Choices, describes levels of prevention as a framework to guide policies that directly affect individual-level choices. Examples illustrating these types of policies include educational guidelines, regulations at the point of purchase, and incentives. Chapter 10, Policy and the Obesogenic Environment, focuses on policies that shape the environment to promote or hinder obesity and includes examples from agriculture, trade, the food industry, and the built environment, along with transportation, schools, and worksites. Chapter 11, Cultural and Familial Influences, describes the role of the immediate social context of culture and family in terms of understanding how they influence dietary habits and physical activities. Chapter 12, Social Justice, Health Disparities, and Obesity, describes the role health disparities play in contributing to obesity and explores resiliency and possible solutions.

The last part of the book, Media and Marketing, discusses pervasive marketing influences and how they affect physical activity, dietary choices, and obesity. Chapter 13, Point of Purchase, describes marketing materials and techniques used at the retail point of purchase to stimulate the purchase and consumption of less healthy foods using product, price, placement, and promotion strategies. Chapter 14, Influence of Media and Technology, describes how images of food influence brain activity which, in turn, contributes to dietary habits. This chapter also provides an overview of the advertising typically used to induce purchase and trial of food.

Throughout the book, we provide recommendations couched within an ecologic framework and tailored to individuals, practitioners, policy makers, communities, and interested citizens. The problem of obesity is an excellent example of the complexities of a public health system. Obesity represents a failure at nearly all levels of the system: genetic predisposition for gaining weight; poor choices by individuals; social traditions that celebrate obesogenic behaviors; community design that limits physical activity; policies that provide for plentiful, nutritionally vacuous food choices and sedentary living; and environments that don't support healthy living and accommodate obese individuals. Reversing the obesity epidemic will take coordinated, multilevel, systemic, long-term efforts that may take years. However, it is possible, and it is never too late to take action.

Obesity is a problem that, ultimately, affects us all, yet it also provides a rich learning opportunity. This text does not provide all the answers, but it will help broaden the scope with which we view this complex societal problem. Thank you for your interest and support.

ACKNOWLEDGMENTS

We wish to thank Scherezade Mama for her tireless encouragement and assistance in the preparation of this manuscript and Ashley Medina for her kind assistance with additional preparation of the document. We also thank the numerous undergraduate interns and graduate students who assisted in the background research, as well as the formatting and proofreading of this manuscript: Heather Adamus, Emily Brown, Christen Crayton, Sharnali Das, TaKoya Davis, Roopa Deepti, Depinder Gill, Jacqueline Dinh, Alejandra Hernandez, Angela Ho, Ygnacio Lopez, Tommy McKey, Majeedah Pacha, Marium Raja, Ryan Renaud, Jacqueline Reese-Smith, Michele Rudolphi, Lily Shirazi, Sameer Siddiqi, Syeda Sidrah, Christopher Sunseri, Raj Thaker, Shivangi Vakharia, and Kristin Wolfe. We are also thankful for the support of important colleagues, including Dr. Charles Layne. Finally, we would like to thank our families and friends for their unconditional love and support and for showing us the importance of healthful dietary habits and regular physical activity.

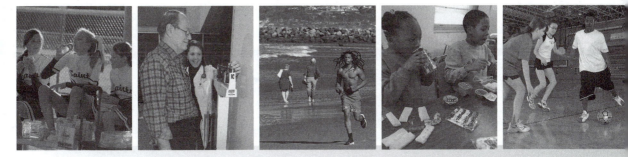

Public Health and Obesity

This first part of the book introduces the concept of the obesogenic environment. Here we define obesity, describe the populations most vulnerable to obesity, discuss the consequences of obesity, and explain the methodologies used to measure obesity. Our obesogenic environment is complex, composed of multiple factors spanning multiple venues, contexts, and sectors. The obesogenic environment has recently been recognized as a factor that contributes to the pervasive lack of physical activity and to eating habits that involve consumption of too much food of poor nutritional quality. The resulting obesity epidemic is now well underway in the United States as well as every other industrialized country. The situation has become so important that U.S. health promoters and researchers have developed a National Physical Activity Plan (2010), building on previous nutritional guidelines and standards. Countries that have been formerly believed to be immune to obesity are facing dramatic increases in its prevalence, particularly among children. It can be hard to understand the scope and causes of the problem. This part of the book sets the stage for the discussion to follow and provides historical background, along with important definitions to give the reader a sense of context. Not all epidemics are reversible, but the obesity epidemic can be, if we reverse the obesogenic environment that created it.

PART

one

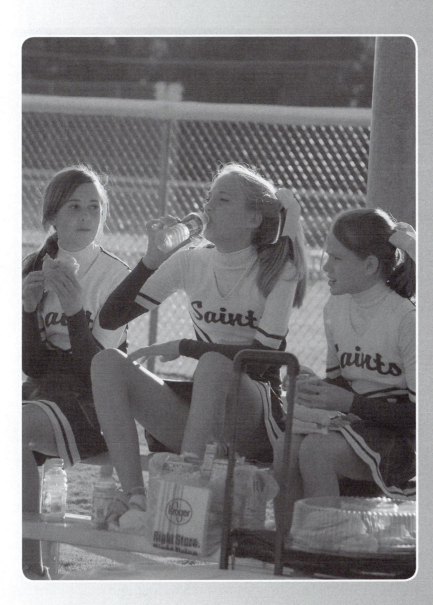

Emergence of the
Obesogenic Environment

Obesity has emerged as the number one public health problem facing the United States as well as many other countries in both the industrialized and developing worlds. Overweight and obesity have historically been a measure of wealth, but in recent times they have come to represent reduced quality of health. Although diet plans and strategies to lose weight are employed multinationally, and many of them are effective in producing weight loss, most are not sustainable. This chapter discusses the historical emergence of obesity and defines some of the etiological factors, external to the individual, that have emerged in recent history. These factors are obesogenic—they create obesity—and represent environmental and social forces that tend to encourage overeating, consumption of unhealthful foods, and physical inactivity, thus promoting weight gain in general. These factors are couched within an ecologic framework that incorporates individual biological and behavioral factors as well as environmental and social forces and their interactions that drive behavior and health outcomes, including obesity.

Obesogenic = obese + genic = something that creates or generates obesity.

Historical Emergence of Obesity as a Public Health Concern

Excess adiposity, or fat, on the body, clinically known as overweight or obesity, has enjoyed a colorful history. In less industrialized times, excess weight signified health and wealth, suggesting that people who were overweight had sufficient, and perhaps excessive, food to eat. Larger body shapes have been immortalized in the past by artists such as Rubens and Renoir, illustrating that the ideal body was one of plenty. Excess adiposity in women, particularly in the breast and hip areas, was considered a symbol of fecundity. The perception of fertility was highly valued in a time where both women and infants died in childbirth and few adults saw their 40th birthday. In men, excess weight was perceived as a sign of wealth and prosperity, suggesting that a man would be a good provider for a family.

In the 20th century, while both longevity and technological innovation increased, preferred body sizes decreased. For example, claims have been made that Marilyn Monroe, one of the greatest sex symbols and models of westernized female beauty of the 20th century, was overweight; however, that is simply not the case. Reports of her height (ranging from 5 feet to 5 feet 5 inches, or 152 to 165 cm) and weight (ranging from approximately 120 to 140 pounds, or 54 to 64 kg) suggest that she had a body mass index close to 23, which is considered nearly ideal by health professionals, and wore a classic size medium dress. She was more slender than her body shape ideal sisters from history, and larger than body shape ideals to come. In the 1970s, in the wake of feminism, androgynous body shapes became very popular; male and female body shape ideals both shrunk to the very slender. It is no coincidence that eating disorders and widespread attention to dieting also emerged about this time. As the 20th century progressed, obesity began to emerge as a widespread public health problem—nearly one in three U.S. adults were obese by the year 2000. Although a combination of factors has contributed to this pendulum swing, many theorists and practitioners believe that an abundance of available food and tremendous technological innovations that reduce physical activity have been prime contributors. We now can get food whenever, wherever, and however we want, and it is easy to spend a lifetime walking no farther than the distance from the garage door to the car and back.

It was also in the late 1970s and early 1980s that public health professionals in the United States began to systematically measure weight as an indicator of health. The prevalence of overweight and obesity has more than doubled among U.S. adults (see figure 1.1) and tripled among U.S. youth. The National Health and Nutrition Examination Survey (NHANES), conducted in the United States, showed that obesity prevalence among U.S. adults aged 20 to 74 increased from 15.0% (in the 1976-1980 survey) to 32.2% (in the 2003-2004 survey) (Flegal, Carroll, Ogden, & Johnson, 2002; Ogden et al., 2006). The problem is emerging in many other countries as well: Estimates range from 1.2 to 1.5 billion overweight or obese on the planet (Ono, Guthold, & Strong, 2005).

The data for youth are particularly disturbing, suggesting that a lifelong struggle with obesity and related health-compromising conditions awaits at least every one in six children born in the United States today. For children

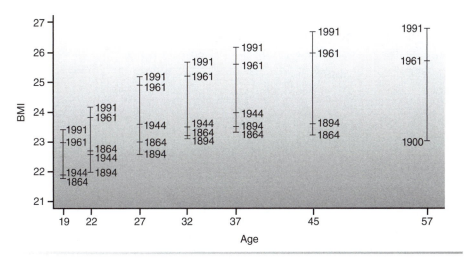

FIGURE 1.1 Historical change in BMI from 1864 to 1991.

Reprinted, by permission, from D.L. Costa and R.H. Steckel, 1997, "Long-term trends in health, welfare, and economic growth in the United States." In *Health and welfare during industrialization*, edited by R.H. Steckel and R. Floud (Chicago: University of Chicago Press). © 1997 by the National Bureau of Economic Research.

ages 2 to 5 years, the prevalence of overweight increased from 5.0% to 13.9%; for those ages 6 to 11 years, prevalence increased from 6.5% to 18.8%; and for those ages 12 to 19 years, prevalence increased from 5.0% to 17.4% (Ogden et al., 2006; Ogden, Carroll, & Flegal, 2008; Ogden, Flegal, Carroll, & Johnson, 2002). A 25-year global analysis of childhood obesity found that although industrialized nations tended to have higher rates of increase, overweight and obesity among children have increased in nearly all countries that collect population data (Wang & Lobstein, 2006).

The Case for an Obesogenic Environment

Because obesity rates have been escalating at annually measurable rates, much research money has been devoted to determining the underlying causes. Despite the world's brightest and best scientific efforts, no single gene or direct pathway explaining obesity has been identified. Numerous genetic factors may contribute to an obesogenic genetic risk profile, but this profile is only an indicator of the potential for someone to gain excess weight under obesogenic conditions. It also happens that most humans share this genetic profile favoring weight gain. There has been no significant genetic shift, mutation, or other biological change in humans in thousands of years. Thus, if the obesogenic genetic risk profile has remained the same in humans since the obesity epidemic began, what has changed?

The answer to this conundrum is both simple and complex. The simple answer is that our environment has changed; the complexity lies in determining the aspects of our environment that have changed to make it obesogenic and how we can reverse the obesogenic environment.

The spectrum of causes of death when we compare today to a century ago is remarkably different in industrialized countries. A century ago, most people died from infectious diseases such as pneumonia or tuberculosis (table 1.1), and most people died young and often relatively quickly. Even if one was overweight or obese, it was less of a concern because the typical health-

TABLE 1.1   Top Causes of Death

1900	2000
1. Influenza and pneumonia	1. Heart disease
2. Tuberculosis	2. Cancer
3. Diarrhea enteritis and ulceration of the intestines	3. Stroke
4. Diseases of the heart	4. Chronic lower respiratory diseases
5. Intracranial lesions	5. Accidents

Adapted from B. Guyer, M.A. Freedman, D.M. Strobino, and E.J. Sondick, 2000, "Annual summary of vital statistics: Trends in the health of Americans during the 20th century," *Pediatrics* 106(6): 1307-1317, and A.H. Mokdad, J.S. Marks, D.F. Stroup, and J.L. Gerberding, 2004, "Actual causes of death in the United States, 2000," *JAMA* 291(10): 1238-1245.

compromising conditions associated with obesity tend to happen later in life, a period in the life cycle that most people did not live long enough to see. In the past century, tremendous scientific advances in microbiology, improved understanding of contagions, and the technological innovation of vaccination have eliminated nearly all deadly infectious diseases from a century ago. Now people live longer lives free from many infectious diseases, and they tend to die much later in the life span from chronic health-compromising conditions that slowly reduce the capacity of one or more organ systems. The top causes of death in industrialized countries are all chronic diseases such as heart disease, cancers, and stroke, for which obesity, lack of physical activity, and dietary habits are strong contributors (Centers for Disease Control and Prevention [CDC] & National Center for Injury Prevention and Control [NCIPC], 2008).

The dramatic shift in causes of death in industrialized society reflects the changes in our environments and resulting lifestyles. Everything has changed. Technological innovation has changed the way our food is grown, prepared, and presented in the retail marketplace. Policies promoting economic growth while yielding to political pressures have changed the food supply. Economic growth and the globalization of the marketplace have increased communication and travel, influencing lifestyle habits and changing available jobs. School policies have changed the types of physical activities taught, if they are taught at all, and the kinds of foods youths learn to love at an early age. Our individual lives have changed. We buy our food already partially or wholly prepared rather than hunt or gather it ourselves. We travel to our jobs and schools by car rather than by foot. Many of us may rely on televisions and computers that bring the world directly to the comfort of our own homes. There are many more examples.

Implementing Policy

The Complex System of Obesity

Obesity is a true complex system problem. The rapid emergence of obesity results from failure at every level in the ecologic milieu, so reversing obesity requires a coordinated effort at every level in the system. Healthy eating and physical activity have to become more appealing, cost efficient, and normative than unhealthful eating and sedentary living, and this is something that cannot be accomplished at a table for one. Partnerships are needed among policy makers, health care professionals, merchants, community organizations, urban planners, farmers, corporations, and scientists to build a more readily available, inexpensive, healthy, and tasty food supply along with many more daily opportunities for physical activity that are more appealing than physical inactivity. Partnerships must think globally, incorporating traditions and cultures from around the world, to prevent the rapid emergence of obesity from taking hold as it has in the United States.

Ecologic Models of Health and the Importance of Supportive Environments

As the prevalence of overweight and obesity has increased, there have been many intervention strategies to reduce weight and maintain weight loss (figure 1.2). These typically focus on the individual person, recommending dietary restrictions and increases in energy expenditure. Although many individually focused interventions have been shown to change behavior (Chen et al., 1998; Collins, Lee, Albright, & King, 2004; Poston et al., 2001; Resnicow et al., 2002), these behavioral changes often are not sustainable in the face of environmental and social forces that shape behavior back to its origin. Up to 50% of those who start a new physical activity program stop within six months (Dishman, 1994; Dishman & Buckworth, 1996). As people lose weight, it gets harder to maintain the level of dietary restriction and physical activity needed for maintaining the lower weight. People may find this new, seemingly abstemious lifestyle too arduous, making it difficult to stay motivated to maintain the weight loss (Klem et al., 2000).

Ecologic models posit that high dropout and low maintenance rates result, in part, from environmental forces that support poor dietary habits and sedentary behavior. Other scholars have suggested that environmental forces may be much larger contributors to health than many realize (Lalonde, 1974). Environmental factors that drive human behavioral patterns are not typically addressed in individually focused programs. For example, in the city of Tokyo, excessive automobile traffic congestion makes driving very slow and unappealing. Many people who own cars, and who could drive around town if they wanted, choose instead to take public transportation because it is much more cost effective and pleasant than driving. It is relatively easy to increase levels of walking when people are already in settings that encourage taking public transportation because people must walk to and from the transit stop. Interventions that incorporate environmental factors are needed (Sallis, Bauman, & Pratt, 1998; Spence & Lee, 2003).

Ecologic models suggest reciprocal relationships among individual, social, and environmental factors (Bronfenbrenner, 1977; Bronfenbrenner, 1979; McLeroy, Bibeau, Steckler, & Glanz, 1988; Sallis et al., 1998; Sallis & Owen, 1997; Spence & Lee, 2003). For example, individual and social factors may contribute to efforts aimed at policy changes that afford construction of a park or improvement of existing facilities. In this example, individual residents of a neighborhood may join together socially to petition the local government to allocate funds to build a park, provide maintenance and security, and promote physical activity programs at the park. If local pressure is strong enough, it may succeed in changing policies that, in turn, improve the lives of individual residents. This is an example of how pressure at one level of an ecologic system can influence change at another level of the ecologic system, which may in turn influence still another level of the ecologic system. Although environments

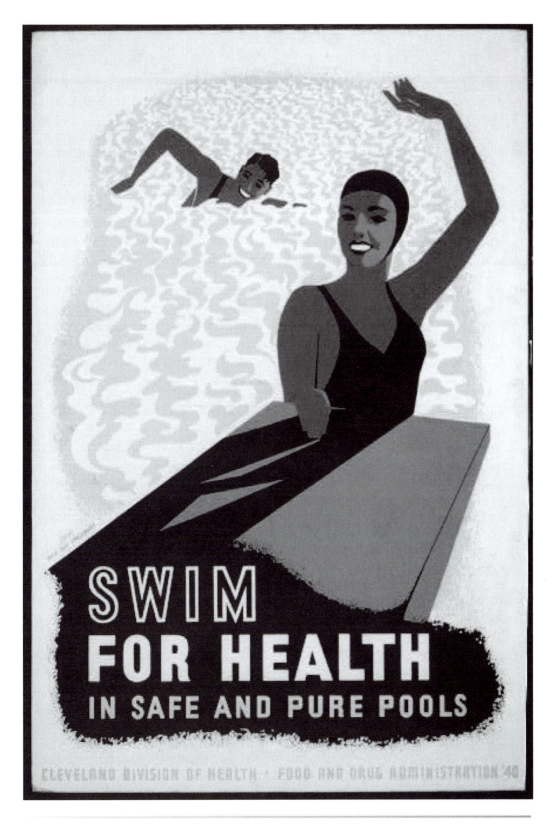

FIGURE 1.2   In the 1940s, the Cleveland Division of Health created this poster promoting swimming as healthy exercise.

Courtesy of the Library of Congress, LC-USZC2-1096.

may change as a result of individual and social factors, this change may take a long time—years or even decades.

A single environmental setting may influence the behavior of many people who live, work, and play within it in a similar way. To use our park example, if a neighborhood has a park that is well maintained and secure, people will use it regardless of social or cultural factors. Children will play, mothers will walk with strollers, others will relax on benches, and exercisers will use the fitness equipment. Thus, ecologic models posit that existing environments influence human behavior similarly, regardless of individual and sociocultural factors.

Ecologic models also suggest that environments shape and modify health behaviors. In the context of physical activity, widely recognized as vital for maintaining a healthy body weight, an environmental factor would be having a safe, pleasant, and convenient place to walk. Along with our park example, it would be helpful to have neighborhood streets that are safe, pleasant, and well connected with lots of goods and services and interesting things to look at for people walking or bicycling by (Eyler, Brownson, Bacak, & Housemann, 2003; Giles-Corti & Donovan, 2003). Having supportive environmental factors contributes to physical activity directly and indirectly. Having an environment that supports physically active transportation and recreation makes it possible for people to choose to be physically active without much thought, because it is easy, fun, and pleasant. In this case, the environment is a direct influence on behavior. The indirect effect occurs because the environment shapes some factor that, in turn, influences behavior. Neighborhoods that have a park nearby and walkable streets may foster positive social and cultural factors (for instance, greater social connectedness and opportunities to interact). The positive social and cultural factors then, in turn, enhance neighborhood safety because walkers feel safe walking in their neighborhood, leading to more physical activity and less obesity.

A number of theorists (Bronfenbrenner, 1977; Bronfenbrenner, 1979; Lee & Cubbin, 2009; McLeroy et al., 1988; Spence & Lee, 2003) have discussed ecologic models in detail. Spence and Lee have conceptualized influences on physical activity, in particular, as micro-, meso-, exo-, and macroenvironmental, with individual-level health behavior and disease states as outcomes. The micro- and macroenvironmental elements may be thought of as relatively static, but these are linked by dynamic meso- and exoenvironmental linkages and processes and influenced by extra-individual forces of change (e.g., technological innovation), and intra-individual factors that are biological and psychological in nature. Although ecologic models somewhat artificially categorize factors, they provide a useful heuristic to investigate how the multiple factors interact and influence physical activity, dietary habits, and obesity.

According to Lee and Cubbin (2009), individual factors (those that are biological, behavioral, or attitudinal) make up a relatively small part of human health (figure 1.3). Numerous microenvironments contribute to behavioral choices. The microenvironment includes the day-to-day environments in which a person lives, works, and plays, like the home, store, church, work, or school. Opportunities for eating and physical activity that are available in these places directly contribute to behavior. For example, after a long morning at church, a social after the service that includes cookies and punch may mean that hungry worshipers may feast on cookies and punch rather

Ecologic milieu = the complex system that encompasses the total ecology of a person, including policy, environmental, social, personal, and biological factors.

than more nutritionally meaningful foods. The child who comes home from school to a refrigerator with fresh fruits and vegetables, already prepared and on a shelf at eye level, will eat more healthfully than the child who comes home to a bag of potato chips and cookies. The microenvironment directly influences choices that can contribute to obesity.

The immediate neighborhood surrounding one's home is another microenvironment that plays an important role in preventing obesity. People who live near public open space, streets with minor traffic, and trees or streets with footpaths or sidewalks and shops are much more likely to achieve recommended levels of physical activity, regardless of their individual income, education, or ethnic background (Giles-Corti & Donovan, 2003). Having a neighborhood grocery store with many high quality and affordable fruits

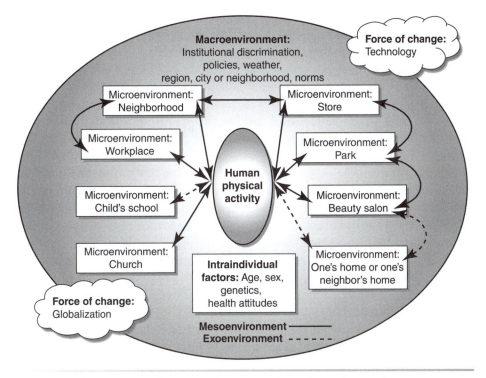

FIGURE 1.3 How multilevel factors influence weight in the ecologic milieu.

Reprinted, by permission, from R.E. Lee and C. Cubbin, 2009, "Striding toward social justice: The ecologic milieu of physical activity," *Exercise and Sports Sciences Reviews* 37(1): 10-17.

and vegetables may increase fruit and vegetable consumption of all residents (Buscher, Martin, & Crocker, 2001; Horgen & Brownell, 2002; Hunt et al., 1990; Morland, Wing, & Diez Roux, 2002; Morland, Wing, Diez Roux, & Poole, 2002), since people tend to make dietary choices based on food that is available and economical (Mooney, 1990).

The mesoenvironment is the dynamic link that connects an individual's microenvironments to each other. This includes both the physical environment linkages and the interactive processes that may occur across microenvironments, such as conversations and other shared experiences. Commuting between work and home represents a mesoenvironment that may differentially influence obesity. If one spends long hours alone in the car commuting to work each day, this decreases time to be physically active, shop, and prepare nutritious food, increases stress, and reduces social connectivity that may also indirectly contribute to obesity.

The exoenvironment is the link that connects an individual's microenvironment with other microenvironments that do not typically include the individual. For example, a child may never visit a parent's workplace, but the circumstances in the work microenvironment may still influence the child's behavior. For example, if the workplace policy promotes physical activity and healthy food choices, the parent who is employed there may begin to adopt more healthy habits, not only at work, but also at home, influencing the child's behavior. The exoenvironment is a connection that can be confusing: It may be difficult to identify the originating microenvironment as well as the affected microenvironments.

The macroenvironment is the broader social context that encompasses the micro-, meso-, and exoenvironments. This includes pervasive influences like institutional discrimination and public policies. Macroenvironmental factors directly influence the behavior of people, above and beyond their individual characteristics. Although the specific mechanisms underlying these relationships are usually not well conceptualized, the associations are reliable and enduring. For example, institutional discrimination lies within the macroenvironmental social structure itself, in comparison to interpersonal discrimination that happens between individuals or internalized discrimination that happens within individuals. Institutional discrimination is usually examined by its results, such as disparities in political and civic representation, access to education, and occupational opportunities, and health behaviors and outcomes. Institutional discrimination is also reflected by the lack of health-promoting urban planning in deprived areas and the converse of greater investment in higher income areas. For example, large national U.S. studies have shown that neighborhoods with higher proportions of black residents have fewer grocery stores and nearly three times the number of liquor stores. Having fewer grocery stores means that there are fewer opportunities to select a wide variety of foods, including fresh fruits and vegetables.

Macroenvironment-level policies centering on transportation and automobile traffic regulation, urban development, and air quality stand to increase the quantity and enhance the quality of the pedestrian and food environments. These policies can directly affect the physical activity and dietary choices of residents at the individual level. For example, traditional suburban neighborhoods may have safe and appealing green space for recreational leisure time activity, but zoning regulations provide few goods and services located near homes. Although neighborhoods may be safe and provide attractive opportunities for physical activity, the physical activity will likely only be done for leisure rather than for active transportation since there are no destinations except other residences available.

The micro-, meso-, exo-, and macroenvironments all contribute to the greater ecologic milieu of the individual. The ecologic milieu refers to everything that contributes to the presence of people of healthy weight who eat nutritious food and perform daily physical activity living in a given environment. All the multilevel environmental influences contribute to promoting an abundant or faltering ecologic milieu. Thus, many people living in the United States may find it difficult to maintain a healthy body weight not because of a particular genetic tendency but rather because their microenvironments (home, school, work) do not support physical activity and healthy dietary choices; their mesoenvironments (commuting) do not allow time or opportunity to promote physical activity or healthy dietary choices; and the macroenvironments (discrimination, institutional policies) do not favor physical activity or healthy eating opportunities. The American ecologic milieu is one of multiple, multilevel obesogenic influences.

The good news is that the ecologic milieu is dynamic, influenced both by external and internal forces, suggesting that change is possible. Pressure for macro system change is manifest as technological innovation, modernization, and globalization. These pressures will differentially affect some groups more or less favorably. Technological innovation occurs with the advent of new methods and protocols for accomplishing formerly human-driven activities with the use of technological advancements—a classic example is the innovation of the computer over the typewriter. Not only does the computer accomplish the same activities as the typewriter, but it also provides other advanced features for reading, writing, and communicating through the use of technology. Technological innovation is functional only to those who can access and use the technology. Globalization means that we have the opportunity to promote and exchange healthy opportunities around the world, with the risk of transmitting our obesogenic environment at the same time.

> Describe how factors at micro, meso, exo, and macro levels in an ecologic system might interact to prevent or promote obesity.

In the face of the ecologic milieu, intraindividual factors—the biology and psychology underlying daily and lifelong experiences—may be less influential for achieving optimal health. There continues to be a perception that physical activity, dietary habits, and related health outcomes such as obesity are guided by individual choice and independent decisions, but this does not acknowledge the pervasive influence of the obesogenic environment in our ecologic milieu. Individual beliefs about physical activity and dietary habits suggest that many people truly believe that if they just had the willpower to stick with a lifestyle change, they, too, could be thinner and healthier. This misperception ignores the reality that individual willpower does not account for the many extraindividual environmental factors that exert influence on the individual. It is true that an individual must have the biological capacity to maintain a healthy weight, in terms of not being physically disabled and having sufficient financial resources to buy healthful food. However, in most cases, actually adopting and maintaining a healthy lifestyle may have very little to do with any individual biology, beliefs, attitudes, or knowledge (Cubbin & Winkleby, 2005; Regan, Lee, Booth, & Reese-Smith, 2006).

GETTING STARTED

❑ Understand the historical emergence of obesity as a public health concern.
❑ Understand why individual motivation alone may not be sufficient to achieve a sustainable healthy body weight.
❑ Describe obesogenic factors in the environment framed within an ecologic model.

Summary

This chapter provides an overview of the emergence of the obesogenic environment. Obesity emerged in the United States as a public health issue toward the beginning of the 1980s, and has been growing measurably ever since. Obesity has now become an international concern that has eclipsed undernutrition in its population reach. Obesity can be considered within an ecologic framework that helps to describe obesogenic environmental, social, and individual influences. Ecologic models of health behavior help us to understand the limitations of focusing solely on individual factors like biological, behavioral, and psychological determinants of obesity. Ecologic models include factors from the built environment, transportation, planning, food security, food availability, technology, and policy, as well as media and other social and cultural influences. Obesity is now considered an epidemic, one that began at least four decades ago. It will take coordinated responses from all levels to reverse our obesogenic environment in order to curb the obesity epidemic and achieve sustained good health for all.

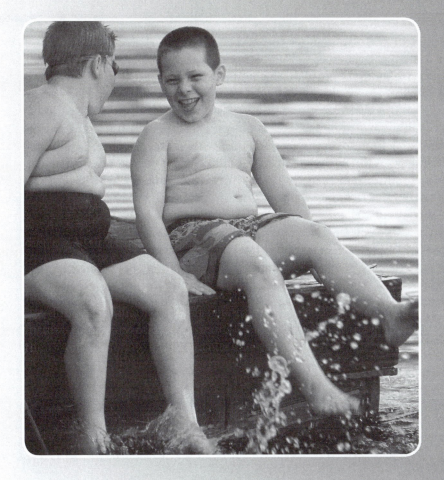

CHAPTER 2

Scope of Obesity

O verweight and obesity have reached epidemic levels globally—well over one billion people are overweight (figure 2.1) (World Health Organization [WHO], 2003). Another way to think about this is that nearly one in five people on the planet or nearly 18% of the world population are overweight or obese (WHO, 2006). It is distressing that overweight has eclipsed undernutrition as a public health concern in developing countries (Misra & Khurana, 2008). In industrialized nations, overweight and obesity have become normative health conditions. For example, the average U.S. adult BMI is equal to 28 (Ogden et al., 2006). About one in three (36.5%) American adults are overweight and another third are obese, meaning that nearly two-thirds of the adult population are at risk for diseases related to overweight and obesity (Ogden et al., 2006). Over half of all states are burdened with an obesity population prevalence over 20% (figure 2.2) (Ogden et al., 2006). Based on measured annual increases in prevalence rates over the past 30 years, it has been predicted that by 2050, everyone in the United States, and possibly the world, will be obese (Bahr, Browning, Wyatt, & Hill, 2009; Wang, Beydoun, Liang, Caballero, & Kumanyika, 2008).

Obesity Defined

Weight status is generally defined by the proportion of weight to height in a simple formula called the body mass index, or BMI. Although there are other definitions of body composition, BMI is the most commonly used definition. (A thorough discussion of body composition and weight status is presented in chapter 3.) The classifications of BMI include the following (National Heart,

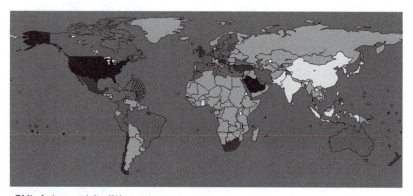

BMI of obese adults (%), most recent

■ ≥ 50.00   ■ 10.00-20.00
■ 40.00-50.00   □ 5.00-10.00
■ 30.00-40.00   □ 0.00-5.00
■ 20.00-30.00   □ no data

FIGURE 2.1   Global BMI prevalence.

Reprinted, by permission, from World Health Organization, 2006, WHO Global Database on Body Mass Index. [Online]. Available: http://apps.who.int/bmi/index.jsp [October 4, 2010].

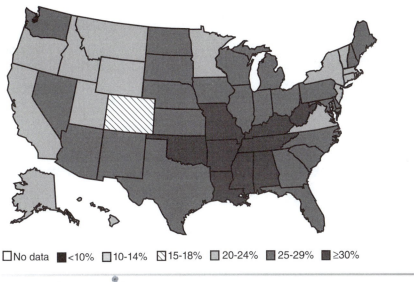

FIGURE 2.2 U.S. obesity prevalence.

Reprinted from Centers for Disease Control and Prevention, 2009, Overweight and obesity: U.S. obesity trends by state 1985-2009. [Online]. Available: www.cdc.gov/obesity/data/trends.html [October 4, 2010].

Lung, and Blood Institute of the National Institutes of Health [NHLBI NIH], 1998):

- Underweight is a weight where there is insufficient weight for a given height for good health or a BMI falling below 18.5 kg/m². Underweight is less common in the industrialized world but is more prevalent in less industrialized nations.

- Normal weight is defined by a BMI that represents a range of weight that is considered healthy for a given height or a BMI falling between 18.5 kg/m² and 24.9 kg/m².

- Overweight is defined as a weight that is too much for a given height or a BMI falling between 25 kg/m² and 29.9 kg/m².

- Obesity is defined as too much weight for a given height for good health or a BMI that meets or exceeds 30 kg/m². Obese weight status is divided into three classes:
  - Class 1 obesity is defined by a BMI falling between 30 kg/m² and 34.9 kg/m².
  - Class 2 obesity is defined by a BMI falling between 35 kg/m² and 39.9 kg/m².
  - Class 3 obesity is defined by a BMI at or above 40 kg/m². Class 3 obesity (sometimes called morbid obesity) is a great health risk because it is difficult for the body to survive in good health with so much extra adiposity. Adiposity is a clinical term used to refer to fat tissue.

TABLE 2.1   **Weight Status, BMI, and Sample Weight Ranges**

Weight status	BMI range (kg/m²)	Weight range for a person 5'4"	Weight range for a person 5'9"	Weight range for a person 6'2"
Underweight	<18.5	<110	<128	<148
Normal weight	18.5-24.9	110-140 lb	128-162 lb	148-186 lb
Overweight	25-29.9	145-169 lb	169-196 lb	194-225 lb
Obese weight class 1	30-34.9	174-204 lb	203-235 lb	233-272 lb
Obese weight class 2	35-39.9	204-227 lb	236-263 lb	273-303 lb
Obese weight class 3	>40	>227 lb	>263 lb	>304 lb

Adapted from U.S. Department of Health and Human Services, 1998, Clinical guidelines on the identification, evaluation, and treatment of overweight and obesity in adults: The evidence report (NIH Publication No. 98-4083). [Online]. Available: www.nhlbi.nih.gov/guidelines/obesity/ob_gdlns.pdf [October 4, 2010].

BMI classifications are summarized in table 2.1.

BMI for children and youth is calculated differently than adults. BMI estimates in children and adolescents account for differences in adiposity, development, and other factors that are unique to developing youth. Children and adolescents are classified as underweight, normal weight, overweight, or obese depending on their weight and height for age and sex.

Causes of Obesity

The majority of obesity in the industrialized world results from too many calories consumed (eating too much) and too few calories expended (physical inactivity). If the number of calories consumed equals the number of calories expended, then weight will stay the same. This is called energy balance. In the case of weight gain or weight loss, there is energy imbalance.

Weight gain and weight loss resulting from energy imbalance are typically very slow processes. It takes the energy associated with 3,500 calories to equal 1 pound (about .5 kg) of weight. This is roughly the number of calories that can be found in 29 slices of bread, 12 cups of ice cream, 10 cheeseburgers, or 36 bananas, and it is about double the number of calories that most dietary guidelines suggest that most people should consume in a day. For most people who are trying to lose weight without medical supervision, guidelines suggest reducing daily caloric consumption by 500 calories, or to about 1,200 to 1,500 calories per day (NHLBI NIH, 1998).

Adiposity = animal fat.

Energy balance = the balance between energy consumed (food eaten) and energy expended (physical activity).

Implementing Policy

Fitness Results on Report Cards

Although obesity has been widely recognized as a public health issue, few members of the general public have a clear understanding of obesity: how it is defined, what the specific guidelines are for prevention and treatment, and who should monitor it. Schools in many states in the United States have fitness standards that children are expected to meet through physical activity and weight status tests. The state of Arkansas has begun publishing weight status (BMI) as part of the grade report cards that are sent to parents from the school on behalf of all public school children. Parents receive a letter explaining that excess body weight is a problem for many children and that it can affect health and learning. Parents are shown a chart illustrating healthy, excessive, and obese weights and an indicator of where their child's weight lies. Parents are advised to contact their doctor for additional screening and information, and they are given general nutrition and physical activity guidelines. Although initially a controversial strategy, the program has become valuable for Arkansas parents, educators, and youth, and the rates of obesity among children in Arkansas have not increased since the program was implemented. This suggests that it may not only increase awareness of the problem but may also help to ameliorate it somewhat (Justus, Ryan, Rockenbach, Katterapalli, & Card-Higginson, 2007).

On the energy expenditure side of the energy balance, 3,500 calories is roughly the amount of energy expended in 6 hours of cycling, 14 hours of walking, 12 hours of dancing, 17 hours of housework, 12 hours of gardening, 8 hours of leisure swimming, 11 hours of golfing, 8 hours of manual lawn mowing, 20 hours of stretching, 18 hours of playing an instrument, or 7 hours of ice skating (American Association of Retired Persons [AARP], 2009). As presented in table 2.2, guidelines for physical activity vary somewhat for adults, but at the minimum suggest at least 30 minutes of moderate intensity physical activity on most days, along with strength training (U.S. Department of Health and Human Services [USDHHS], 2008).

Recommendations for children and youth suggest a minimum of 60 minutes of physical activity for most days of the week. The published guidelines also generally suggest that additional health benefits can be achieved by increasing the duration and intensity of physical activity. Several agencies have also suggested that people who are trying to lose weight or maintain weight loss should get at least double or more of the amount of physical activity recommended for general health guidelines.

A relatively small variation in dietary habits or physical activity can lead to weight gain or weight loss if nothing else changes. For example, between the ages of 25 and 55, it has been estimated that the average American adult

TABLE 2.2   **Guidelines for Physical Activity**

Recommendations	CDC	ACSM	IOM	WHO	AHA
Adults—healthy weight	Do 150 minutes of moderately intense physical activity a week, and 2 or more days of muscle strengthening activities.	Do moderately intense cardio 30 minutes a day, 5 days a week. *Or* do 20 minutes of vigorously intense cardio 3 days a week. *And* do 8 to 10 strength-training exercises, 8 to 12 repetitions of each exercise, twice a week.	Do at least one hour of moderately intense physical activity each day.	Do 30 minutes of moderately intense physical activity 5 days per week, or 20 minutes of vigorous-intensity physical activity 3 days per week and 8-10 muscular strengthening exercises (8-12 repetitions) at least 2 days per week.	Do moderate-to vigorous-intensity aerobic activity for at least 30 minutes on most days of the week at 50–85 percent of the maximum heart rate.
Adults—weight loss	Do 300 minutes of moderately intense physical activity a week, and 2 or more days of muscle strengthening activities.	Do moderately intense cardio 60 to 90 minutes a day, 5 days a week. *And* do 8 to 10 strength-training exercises, 8 to 12 repetitions of each exercise, twice a week.			
Children—healthy weight	Do 60 or more minutes of physical activity a day.	Do 60 minutes or up to several hours of physical activity each day of the week.	Do at least one hour of moderately intense physical activity each day.	Do 60 minutes of moderately to vigorously intense physical activity each day that is developmentally appropriate and involves a variety of activities.	Do at least 60 minutes of moderate to vigorous physical activity every day.

Adapted from Centers for Disease Control and Prevention, 2010; American College of Sports Medicine and the American Heart Association, 2007; American College of Sports Medicine, 2006; Institute of Medicine of the National Academies of Science, 2002; World Health Organization, 2010; and American Heart Association, 2010.

gains one pound of fat mass per year and loses one-half pound of muscle mass (Forbes, 1999). It is easy to see how this could happen. Simply eating 100 calories extra per day, and not expending those calories through a small increase in physical activity, could cause a 1-pound gain of fat per year. Eating 100 calories is roughly equivalent to an extra egg, banana, or slice of bread, or about an ounce of potato chips. Meanwhile, expending 100 calories is roughly equivalent to 1 mile (1.6 km) of running or walking briskly, 20 minutes of moderate swimming, 15 minutes of casual basketball, or 30 minutes of bowling. It is easy to see how many of us seem to wake up one morning and realize that, ever so gradually, we have become overweight or obese.

Although BMI is an important indicator of potential health risks associated with being overweight or obese, there are other important indicators health care professionals should consider. These include waist circumference (because abdominal fat is a predictor of risk for obesity-related diseases) and other risk factors, such as family history, or other risk behaviors, such as tobacco use (figure 2.3). Although having a family history can predispose someone toward developing certain diseases associated with obesity, environmental factors and lifestyle factors contribute about 50% of the risk toward actually developing the disease (Satcher, 2001). It is a great benefit to people who have a family history of obesity-related diseases to maintain a healthy body weight to cut their own personal risk of developing disease in half.

Vulnerable Populations

Some subgroups of the population tend to be more vulnerable to obesity than others. The causal mechanisms behind most of these particular vulnerabilities are not well understood; however, there are well-documented differences. In general, people of color, women, disabled populations, and people with less education, lower incomes, and fewer capital resources tend to be more vulnerable to developing obesity, even after accounting for potential differences in BMI measurement. As well, obesity tends to track in families: Children of obese parents are at greater risk of becoming obese themselves (Pinot de Moira, Power, & Li, 2010; Whitaker, Wright, Pepe, Seidel, & Dietz, 1997). These children are likely at higher risk for both genetic and behavioral reasons. A number of predisposing genes may be transmitted from one generation to the next, and parenting and child-feeding practices may also contribute to these vulnerabilities (Vos & Welsh, 2010).

Overweight and obesity rates tend to be higher among populations of color compared to whites in the United States. The problem is particularly evident in black populations: Nearly 70% of black adults are overweight or obese, compared to only 60% of white adults (table 2.3 on p. 23). In Texas, 69% of black adults are overweight or obese compared to 60% of white adults (CDC, 2008).

Disparities in overweight and obesity in the United States, along with many other industrialized nations, are also evident among lower socioeconomic status populations, and people with lower educational attainment, income, or capital resources (Moore, Hall, Harper, & Lynch, 2010). The data presented in table 2.4 on page 23, from the most recent National Health and Nutrition Examination

My Personal Profile

Name: _____

Today's date: _____

Age: _____

Height (in.): _____

Weight (lb.): _____ Waist size (in.): _____

BMI: Use the BMI chart on page 12 or use this equation:

$$\frac{wt\ (lb.)}{Height\ (in.)\ x\ height\ (in.)} \times 703 = \rule{5cm}{0.4pt}$$

BMI ranges:

- < 18.5 = underweight
- 18.5–24.9 = normal weight
- 25–29.9 = overweight
- > 30 = obese

My BMI indicates that I am: (Please circle)
underweight   normal weight   overweight   obese

My risk factors are: (Please circle)

- high blood pressure (hyper tension)
- high LDL cholesterol ("bad" cholesterol)
- low HDL cholesterol ("good" cholesterol)
- high triglycerides
- high blood glucose (sugar)
- family history of premature heart disease
- physical inactivity
- cigarette smoking

My physical activity level is: (Please circle)
sedentary   moderately active   active

- *Sedentary* means a lifestyle that includes only the light physical activity associated with typical day-to-day life.
- *Moderately* active means a lifestyle that includes physical activity equivalent to walking about 1.5 to 3 miles per day at 3 to 4 miles per hour, in addition to the light physical activity associated with typical day-to-day life.
- *Active* means a lifestyle that includes physical activity equivalent to walking more than 3 miles per day at 3 to 4 miles per hour, in addition to the light physical activity associated with typical day-to-day life

A healthy weight range for my height is: (Based on the BMI chart) _____

Estimated daily calorie needs, my goal: _____

FIGURE 2.3 Use this worksheet to help your clients easily determine their BMI, risk factors, and activity level. For the BMI chart, see page 12 of the source publication.

Reprinted from U.S. Department of Health and Human Services, Office of Disease Prevention and Health Promotion, 2005, *A healthier you: Based on the Dietary Guidelines for Americans* (Washington, DC: U.S. Department of Health and Human Services), 89.

TABLE 2.3   Overweight and Obesity in the United States by Race

	White	Black	Latino	Other	Multiracial
All adults (age adjusted, 20 years and over) by race in 2006					
Overweight (%)	36.8	35.1	37.7	31.9	34.3
Obese (%)	24.2	36.7	25.5	18.7	27.0
Texas adults (age adjusted, 20 years and over) by race in 2008					
Overweight (%)	35.6	34.3	41.8	32.2	NSD
Obese (%)	26.3	38.8	32.9	13.1	NSD

Adapted from Ogden et al., 2007, and Centers for Disease Control and Prevention, 2008.

Survey (NHANES), indicate that those in poverty (below 100% of poverty level) have lower rates of overweight but higher rates of obesity compared to higher income brackets (Ogden, Carroll, McDowell, & Flegal, 2007). Obesity also increases as educational attainment and available capital resources decrease. Many believe that those in poverty with low educational attainment may not have the personal resources or knowledge to maintain a healthy body weight; however, the relationship is more complex than this simple individual level explanation.

What is the true cost of obesity? How is this defined for individuals? How is this defined for societies?

Later in this book, possible putative mechanisms for this relationship are offered that emphasize factors throughout the ecologic milieu.

Women tend to have lower rates of overweight (27.4%) and higher rates of obesity (34%) compared to men (40.5% and 30.2%, respectively) (Ogden, Carroll, McDowell, & Flegal, 2007). This pattern of overweight status by sex is also seen throughout the world (Moore, Hall, Harper, & Lynch, 2010), reflecting biological sex differences in body composition and additional weight often gained (and not lost) as a result of pregnancy. One out of every four women, compared to two out of every five men, are overweight in the United States.

TABLE 2.4   Overweight and Obesity in U.S. Adults by Poverty

	Percent of poverty level		
	<100%	100%–200%	200%+
Overweight (%)	29.0	31.6	35.5
Obese (%)	34.9	34.6	30.6

Age adjusted 20 years and over.

Adapted from Ogden et al., 2007.

Health Risks Associated With Overweight and Obesity

The BMI weight status classification into underweight, normal weight, overweight, and obese identifies ranges of weight that have been shown to increase the likelihood of certain diseases and other health-compromising conditions in numerous clinical studies. On average, across many studies, the ideal BMI for reducing health risk is somewhere between 22 and 23 (Kannel, D'Agostino, & Cobb, 1996). Health risk increases in people who are underweight and again as people transition from overweight to obese weight status categories. This forms a J-shape distribution, suggesting that too little weight and too much weight both present health risks (figure 2.4). There truly is an energy balance that best promotes health. Many health-compromising conditions have been associated with overweight and obesity. These include coronary heart disease, stroke, hypertension, dyslipidemia, gallbladder disease, osteoarthritis, sleep apnea, and respiratory problems. Also, numerous cancers are associated with overweight and obesity, including endometrial, breast, and colon cancers (NHLBI NIH, 1998).

At least 4 of the top 10 leading causes of death identified by the U.S. Department for Health and Human Services are directly caused by or indirectly associated with obesity. The risk of death from all causes increases by over 100% among the obese. For specific diseases, the situation is even bleaker. Death from heart disease—the most common cause of death in the United States—increases over 200% among the overweight and well over 300% among the obese. Death from type 2 diabetes increases by 3,000% among the obese (Gibbs, 1996). Additionally, obesity has become the top cause of cancer in

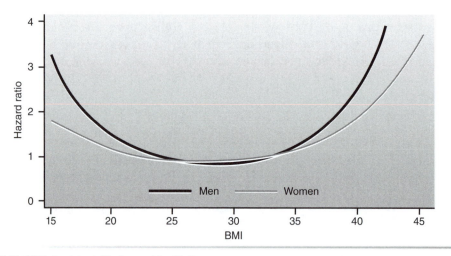

FIGURE 2.4   Mortality hazard by BMI.

Reprinted, by permission, from A. Zajacova, 2008, Shape of the BMI-mortality association by cause of death, using generalized additive models: NHIS 1986-2002 (Population Studies Center, University of Michigan Institute for Social Research, Report 08-639).

the United States. Annually measurable increases in obesity, and the resulting uncontrolled growth in expenditures, contribute to economic disaster for many, including increases in personal and federal debt. Over half of all bankruptcies in America are a direct result of unpaid medical expenses, many of which result from diseases that are due, in part, to obesity. Over 280,000 American deaths and $147 billion in medical expenses are attributed to obesity and obesity-related conditions each year. These expenses reflect direct costs of obesity, including preventive, diagnostic, and treatment services, as well as indirect costs, including morbidity and mortality. Over half of these expenses are paid for by taxpayers through Medicare and Medicaid. Obesity-related medical bills cost every taxpayer about $180 per year, regardless of whether the taxpayer is obese (Finkelstein, Fiebelkorn, & Wang, 2003). From an employer's perspective, medical costs are 77% higher for obese employees than healthy employees, costing employers over $8,000 per person per year. In addition to increased medical costs, obese employees have a higher number of work limitations, leading to poor productivity (Leade Health, 2006).

Social and Psychological Costs of Obesity

In addition to physical health costs associated with obesity, there are significant social and psychological costs. These span various domains affecting individual occupational achievement, educational attainment, health care, and relationships with peers and romantic partners; they have also shaped many societal trends. The obese are less likely than their nonobese counterparts to be employed. Obese people also tend to make less money for the same work (Baum & Ford, 2004; Cawley, 2000; Cawley, 2004; Morris, 2007). It is unclear to what extent this differential is driven by greater prevalence of related health-compromising conditions that limit productivity or are due to discrimination against hiring and promoting the obese. There is very limited evidence to support discrimination in education, perhaps because the more historically progressive academy may be less concerned with appearance compared to other venues. However, traditional classroom settings may be uncomfortable for the obese, because the desks might not accommodate individuals with larger body mass. Some industries, such as the airlines, have begun to recognize the need for larger seats and strategies to accommodate larger people; however, this is not universal. Perhaps most disturbing is the finding from a comprehensive international review of studies of health care providers from a range of disciplines (doctors, nurses, medical students, and dietitians) that found that most providers tend to have negative attitudes toward the obese, which may hamper productive preventive care, weight gain intervention, and treatment (Puhl & Heuer, 2009).

There is some evidence to suggest that the obese may perceive discrimination in romantic partnerships and friendships, although research and data to support these claims are limited. On the other hand, it is often difficult to measure and quantify sensitive issues related to the stigma of obesity, and future work is needed in order to understand this issue. It is clear that the obese who perceive greater weight bias tend to be more susceptible to low self-esteem, depressive symptoms, body image concerns, and maladaptive eating behaviors. Few effective intervention strategies have been identified for coping with these psychosocial concerns (Puhl & Heuer, 2009).

It is interesting to note societal trends that have changed as a result of larger body sizes becoming normative. Sports arenas are now built with more capacious seating to accommodate wider fans (Patton, 1999). Airlines now budget more average weight per passenger, since the average passenger is now typically 10 pounds (5 kg) heavier than when the industry originated (Phillips, 2003). Ready-to-wear clothing sizes have changed: A size 14 dress made in 1940 would now be a size 10 (Nifong & Gerhard, 1999). Health care devices have been modified to accommodate an obese population. Needles used for injections are now typically longer to penetrate a larger subcutaneous fat mass, and blood pressure cuffs and wheelchairs are larger to fit larger bodies (Nagourney, 2000). Still other data suggest that obesity is a burden to the planet because of the greater demand on the food supply and costs associated with feeding and transporting overweight and obese people who eat and weigh more than lean people (Himmelstein, Warren, Thorne, & Woolhandler, 2005). The consequences of obesity are evident across a wide range of physical, social, psychological, and societal dimensions.

GETTING STARTED

❏ Describe the causes of obesity related to energy balance.
❏ Identify the populations most vulnerable to obesity for both youth and adults.
❏ Describe the individual and societal risks and burdens associated with obesity.

Summary

Although in these days of heightened homeland security much attention has been focused on terrorism and war, in reality a bigger threat to national security is obesity (Lee, 2009). The escalating costs related to health care, loss of productivity, and other limitations are very worrisome and threaten economic and political stability. Overweight and obesity is typically defined by the body mass index that signifies too much weight for a given height. Most cases of overweight and obesity result from excess calories consumed and too few calories expended; thus, obesity is believed to be preventable. The trajectory toward obesity is slow and insidious. Although some population groups are more vulnerable to obesity than others, no single demographic factor reduces the risk of obesity sufficiently to reduce the overall burden of obesity for the population. Overweight and obesity lead to numerous health-compromising conditions and may hamper medical care, as many health care providers have unfavorable attitudes toward the obese. There are significant individual and societal consequences of obesity. The problem of obesity affects everyone and is a significant problem that can be solved only with broad-based efforts incorporating multilevel, diversely focused strategies.

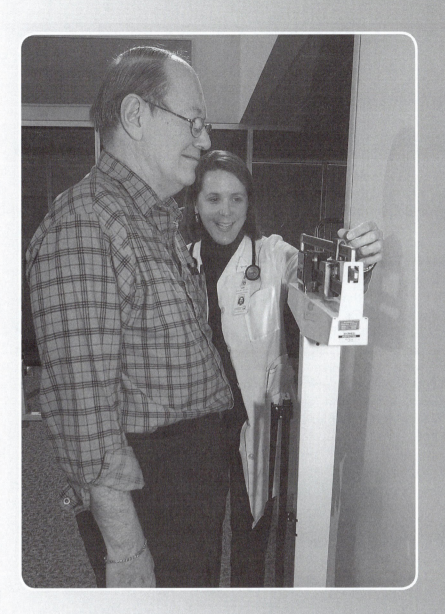

CHAPTER 3

Body Composition
Measurements

ody composition refers to the components of the body, such as fat, lean tissue, and bone. Accurately measuring body composition is important because overweight and obesity are risk factors for a number of adverse health conditions. As a result of this association, health professionals in a variety of settings rely on accurate measures of body composition. For example, health practitioners rely on accurate measures to identify individuals to treat for overweight and obesity, and whether to screen for additional health-compromising conditions. Researchers and public health professionals rely on accurate measures to track the prevalence of overweight and obesity, to understand their determinants, and to determine the effectiveness of intervention efforts. Thus, accurately measuring body composition is extremely important.

Methods of measuring body composition can be categorized in several ways. For the purposes of this chapter, methods of measuring body composition are divided into field methods and laboratory methods. Field methods rely on portable equipment that can be used anywhere and consist of body mass index (BMI), circumferences, skinfold measurement, and bioelectrical impedance analysis (BIA). Laboratory methods rely on equipment permanently established in one location and consist of underwater weighing and dual-energy X-ray absorptiometry (DXA). Although there are many other methods of measuring body composition, these were chosen to discuss because they are most often used by practitioners and researchers. Furthermore, because field methods are primarily used in public health and community settings, whereas laboratory methods are primarily used in clinical and research settings, this chapter primarily focuses on field methods.

This chapter provides background information on the rationale, strengths, and limitations of each body composition method to assist the reader in choosing the most appropriate method. Choosing the most appropriate method for measuring body composition typically depends on the cost associated with it, the population that will be tested, the amount of time required to measure a participant, and the invasiveness of the method. All of these factors must be considered when determining which method is most appropriate under any given circumstance.

Field Methods

The following sections discuss, in turn, body mass index (BMI), waist circumference, the skinfold measurement, and bioelectrical impedance analysis (BIA), focusing on the rationale behind their use, their applicability to different population subgroups, and their strengths and limitations.

Body Mass Index

Body mass index (BMI), a ratio of body weight to height, is a screening tool for categorizing adults as underweight, normal weight, overweight, and obese (CDC, 2007b), and children and adolescents as underweight, healthy weight, overweight, and obese (CDC, 2007c). The following sections describe how to measure and categorize BMI.

Measuring BMI in Adults   In adults, BMI is used to classify individuals into categories that are not age- or sex-specific (see table 2.1 on page 18 for these categories). BMI is calculated using the following equation (CDC, 2007b):

$$\text{BMI} = \frac{\text{Weight in kilograms}}{\text{Height in meters}^2} \tag{3.1}$$

Let's practice calculating and categorizing BMI in adults.

EXAMPLE 1

Calculate and categorize BMI for a 32-year-old male who is 5 feet 9 1/2 in. tall and weighs 259 lb.

Step 1: Convert weight from pounds to kilograms.

1 kg = 2.2046 lb

259 lbs = 117.48 kg

Step 2: Convert height from feet and inches to meters.

1 ft = 12 in.

1 in. = 0.0254 m

5 ft 9 1/2 in. = 69.5 in. = 1.765 m

Step 3: Calculate BMI.

Weight in kilograms = 117.48

Height in meters = 1.765

$$\text{BMI} = \frac{117.48}{(1.765)^2} = 37.71 \text{ kg/m}^2$$

Step 4: Categorize BMI.

BMI of 37.71 kg/m² = obese

Measuring BMI in Children and Adolescents   In children and adolescents, an age- and sex-specific BMI percent is calculated using the same equation used in adults (equation 3.1) (CDC, 2007b). An age- and sex-specific BMI z-score is then calculated using the following equation (3.2) (CDC, 2007a):

$$\text{z-score} = \frac{\left[(X \div M)^{\text{L}}\right] - 1}{LS} \tag{3.2}$$

In this equation, X is the BMI value calculated from equation 3.1, and L, M, and S are age- and sex-specific parameters that can be found on the CDC Web site (CDC, 2007a). Last, an age- and sex-specific BMI z-score is converted to an age- and sex-specific BMI percentile, which is then used to classify children and adolescents into a BMI category (table 3.1) (CDC, 2007c).

TABLE 3.1   BMI Percentile Classification for Children and Adolescents

BMI percentile	BMI percentile classification
<5th percentile	Underweight
5th percentile to <85th percentile	Healthy weight
85th to <95th percentile	Overweight
≥95th percentile	Obese

Adapted from Centers for Disease Control and Prevention, 2009, Healthy weight—It's not a diet, it's a lifestyle! About BMI for children and teens. [Online]. Available: www.cdc.gov/healthyweight/assessing/bmi/childrens_bmi/about_childrens_bmi.html [October 4, 2010].

Let's practice calculating and categorizing BMI percentile in children and adolescents.

EXAMPLE 2

Calculate and categorize BMI percentile for a female, 11 years and 3 1/4 months old, who is 5 ft 1 1/2 in. tall and weighs 137 lb.

Step 1: Convert weight from pounds to kilograms.

　　1 kg = 2.2046 lb

　　137 lb = 62.143 kg

Step 2: Convert height from feet and inches to meters.

　　1 ft = 12 in.

　　1 in. = 0.0254 m

　　5 feet 1 1/2 in. = 61.5 in. = 1.562 m

Step 3: Calculate BMI.

　　Weight in kilograms = 62.143

　　Height in meters = 1.562

$$BMI = \frac{62.143}{(1.562)^2} = 25.47 \text{ kg/m}^2$$

Step 4: Calculate an age- and sex-specific BMI z-score.

$X = 25.47$; $M = 17.625698688$; $L = -2.022817914$; $S = 0.1452061381$

$$\text{BMI z-score} = \frac{\left[(25.47 \div 17.625698688)^{-2.022817914}\right] - 1}{(-2.022817914)(0.1452061381)} = 1.79$$

Step 5: Convert the age- and sex-specific BMI z-score to an age- and sex-specific BMI percentile using a standard normal distribution table found in most statistics textbooks and online.

BMI z-score of 1.79 = 96th percentile

Step 6: Categorize age- and sex-specific BMI percentile.

96th percentile = obese

In addition to using the equations and table just presented, the CDC has growth charts that can be downloaded and used for categorizing BMI percentile (CDC, 2007c). The process is relatively simple and involves selecting the appropriate chart, calculating BMI, and plotting BMI against age on the chart. BMI percentile categorization is then determined by identifying where on the chart the information was plotted; areas of the chart correspond to underweight, healthy weight, overweight, and obese. In addition, the CDC, several hospitals, and various organizations have BMI percentile calculators available on their Web sites where the BMI percentiles can be calculated and categorized when the appropriate information is entered.

Strengths and Limitations   On a population level, BMI has several strengths and few limitations. Compared to other methods of measuring body composition, BMI is fairly easy to measure. For example, the skinfold method requires a considerable amount of training and knowledge of anatomy. BMI does not require in-depth knowledge or training because height, weight, age, and sex are relatively easy to measure and collect. In addition, because height and weight can be collected quickly, a large number of participants can be measured in a short time. For example, it may take 2 or 3 minutes to measure and collect the information needed to calculate and categorize BMI, but as many as 10 minutes for other methods, such as the skinfold method and dual-energy X-ray absorptiometry (DXA).

There are other strengths in using the BMI method. Unlike other methods, BMI does not intrude on participant privacy; measuring height and weight and collecting sex and age information are not invasive. For example, the skinfold method requires participants to remove some of their clothing, such as men removing their shirts, and for assessors to pinch their subcutaneous fat at various locations. Although the costs associated with measuring BMI may seem high, compared to other methods they are actually quite low. For instance, the equipment needed to measure height and weight may cost as much as $300, while bioelectrical impedance analysis (BIA) equipment may cost as much as $1,500. A final strength is that BMI is not sex specific in adults. While the equations used to measure body composition with the skinfold method in adults are sex specific, the BMI equation is not.

A limitation of BMI is that although there is a strong correlation between BMI and percent body fat (Gallagher et al., 1996), BMI does not directly measure body fat. As a result, someone may have a BMI that identifies them as overweight or obese even if they do not have excess body fat. For example, highly trained athletes may have BMIs that are classified as overweight when they may actually have a high amount of musculature and low body fat. A concern that has recently been noted is that the BMI values used to define over-weight and obesity systematically overestimate the prevalence of overweight and obesity among black men and women and underestimate the prevalence among Asian and Latina women (Jackson, Ellis, McFarlin, Sailors, & Bray, 2009). This has important implications because some population groups may be at a higher risk for health-compromising conditions related to overweight and obesity than their BMI value would suggest.

Waist Circumference

The rationale behind using circumferences as a body composition measure-ment is that the distribution of a person's body fat is an important indicator of health risk (Rexrode et al., 1998; Whaley, 2006). Although many circum-ferences are used in body composition measurement, this section focuses on waist circumference. In adults, waist circumference can be used alone, in combination with BMI, and in combination with hip circumference to create a waist-to-hip ratio. The sections that follow discuss the use of waist circum-ference alone and in combination with BMI.

Measuring Waist Circumference   Waist circumference is measured at the narrowest part of the torso, above the umbilicus and below the xiphoid process, approximately at the iliac crest (figure 3.1) (Whaley, 2006). When measuring waist circumference, it's important for the tape measure to be placed directly on the body, rather than over clothing, which could introduce error in the measurement. However, keep in mind that this will require participants to lift their shirts high enough to allow the assessor to access the necessary area. In addition, the tape measure needs to be level, not elevated at one side of the body. The assessor needs to sit or kneel at the participant's side rather than in front or behind the participant, which may make the person feel uncom-fortable. The assessor should ask a colleague for assistance rather than wrap arms around the participant to get the tape measure around the waist. When possible, assessors and participants should be of the same sex. Finally, the standard protocol is to take multiple measurements and to use the average of those measurements. However, if the measurements differ considerably, make sure that proper measurement techniques are being used.

When used alone, a waist circumference greater than 102 cm (40 in.) in men and 88 cm (35 in.) in women indicates an increased risk for a number of adverse health conditions ("Executive summary of the clinical guidelines on the identification, evaluation, and treatment of overweight and obesity in adults," 1998; "Executive summary of the third report of the national cholesterol education program (NCEP) expert panel on detection, evaluation, and treatment of high blood cholesterol in adults (Adult Treatment Panel III)," 2001). Waist circumference can also be used in combination with BMI to determine one's risk for type 2 diabetes, hypertension, and cardiovascular disease ("Executive summary of the clinical guidelines on the identification, evaluation, and treatment of overweight and obesity in adults," 1998).

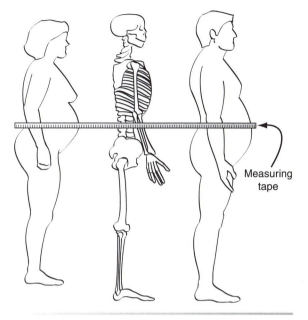

FIGURE 3.1   Measurement sites for waist circumference.

Let's practice by categorizing the waist circumference and BMI of an adult male.

EXAMPLE 3

What is the disease risk of a 36-year-old male who is 6 ft 1 1/2 in. tall, weighs 210 lb, and has a waist circumference of 108 cm?

Step 1: Convert weight from pounds to kilograms.

1 kg = 2.2046 lb
250 lbs = 113.40 kg

Step 2: Convert height from feet and inches to meters.

1 ft = 12 in.
1 in. = 0.0254 m
6 ft 1 1/2 in. = 73.5 in. = 1.867 m

Step 3: Calculate BMI.

Weight in kilograms = 113.40

Height in meters = 1.867

$$BMI = \frac{113.40}{(1.867)^2} = 32.53 \text{ kg/m}^2$$

Step 4: Categorize disease risk.

A male with a BMI of 32.53 kg/m^2 and a waist circumference of 108 cm has a very high risk.

Strengths and Limitations of Waist Circumference Compared to other methods of measuring body composition, waist circumference is fairly easy to measure. Although measuring waist circumference requires some knowledge of anatomy, it does not require as much training or knowledge as other methods, such as the skinfold method. In addition, because waist circumference can be measured quickly, this method allows a large number of participants to be assessed in a short time. However, waist circumference can be invasive and uncomfortable for the participant. As previously mentioned, people being measured will have to lift their shirts high enough to allow the assessor to accurately measure their waists, potentially causing them to feel uncomfortable or embarrassed. A second limitation is that waist circumference does not measure body composition. However, it is a common tool for assessing a person's risk for developing adverse health conditions.

Skinfold Method

The rationale behind the skinfold method is that the amount of subcutaneous fat a person has is proportional to the total amount of body fat (Whaley, 2006).

Implementing Policy

Waist Circumferences in Japan

In an effort to reduce the prevalence of overweight, obesity, and their adverse health conditions, Japan passed a national law in 2008 requiring companies and local governments to measure the waists (i.e., waist circumference) of individuals between the ages of 40 and 74 years during their annual checkups (Onishi, 2008). As part of this national law, the maximum waist circumference allowed was set at 33.5 inches (85 cm) for men and 35.4 inches (90 cm) for women. In an effort to achieve its goal of reducing the prevalence of overweight by 10% over the next four years and by 25% over the next seven years, significant financial penalties will be imposed on companies and local governments that fail to meet specific target goals. As an example of the financial significance of this national law, NEC, Japan's largest maker of personal computers, stated that if it failed to meet its targets, it could incur as much as $19 million in penalties (Onishi, 2008).

Measuring body composition with the skinfold method varies according to the age of the population under investigation because children, adolescents, and adults are measured differently. For example, not only are the equations and measurement sites different, but there are also several issues to consider when working with children and adolescents.

Measuring Skinfolds in Adults In adults, the skinfold method is a two-step process in which body density and percent of body fat are calculated. There are two sets of sex-specific equations for calculating body density in adults. The first set of equations includes age and the sum of three skinfold sites (equations 3.3 for men and 3.4 for women). The three skinfold sites are the chest, abdomen, and thigh in men (Jackson & Pollock, 1978), and the triceps, suprailium, and thigh in women (Jackson, Pollock, & Ward, 1980).

Body density = $1.10938 - 0.0008267 \, (\Sigma 3) + 0.0000016 \times (\Sigma 3)^2$
$- 0.0002574 \, (\text{age})$

($\Sigma 3$ = chest + abdomen + thigh)

($R = 0.905$; *SE* body density = 0.0077) (3.3)

Body density = $1.0994921 - 0.0009929 \, (\Sigma 3) + 0.0000023 \, (\Sigma 3)^2$
$- 0.0001392 \, (\text{age})$

($\Sigma 3$ = Triceps + suprailium + thigh)

($R = 0.842$; *SE* body density = 0.0086) (3.4)

The second set of equations includes age and the sum of seven skinfold sites (equations 3.5 for men and 3.6 for women) (Jackson & Pollock, 1978; Jackson et al., 1980). The seven skinfold sites, which are the same for men and women, are the chest, axilla, triceps, subscapula, abdomen, suprailium, and thigh (figure 3.2 *a-g*). Unfortunately, a detailed description of the anatomical locations of these sites is beyond the scope of this chapter. However, this information can be found in many sources that focus exclusively on body composition measurement and exercise testing (Baumgartner et al., 2003; Whaley, 2006).

Body density = $1.112 - 0.00043499 \, (\Sigma 7) + 0.00000055 \, (\Sigma 7)^2$
$- 0.00028826 \, (\text{age})$

($\Sigma 7$ = chest + axilla + triceps + subscapula + abdomen + suprailium + thigh)

($R = 0.902$; *SE* body density = 0.0078) (3.5)

Body density = $1.0970 - 0.00046971 \, (\Sigma 7) + 0.00000056 \, (\Sigma 7)^2$
$- 0.00012828 \, (\text{age})$

($\Sigma 7$ = chest + axilla + triceps + subscapula + abdomen + suprailium + thigh)

($R = 0.852$; *SE* body density = 0.0083) (3.6)

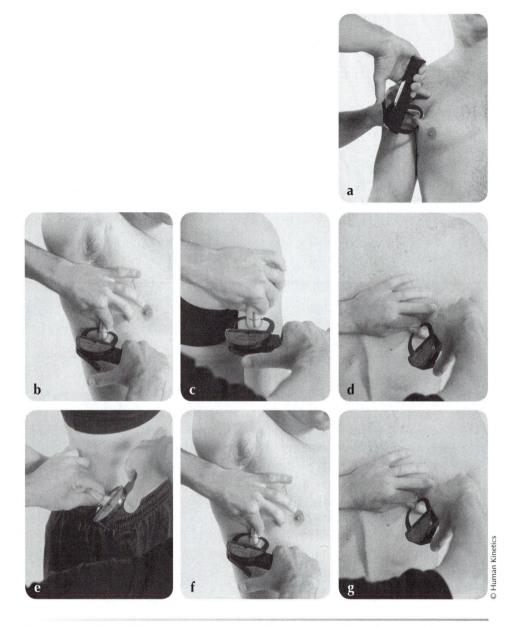

FIGURE 3.2 Skinfold sites for *(a)* chest, *(b)* axilla, *(c)* triceps, *(d)* subscapula, *(e)* abdomen, *(f)* suprailium, and *(g)* thigh.

Finally, because of the high correlation between the sum of three and seven skinfolds, and because they have similar correlations with percent body fat, the three-site skinfold equations are used more often because they save time and intrude less on participant privacy. Let's practice calculating body density using the three skinfold site equations (example 4).

EXAMPLE 4

Calculate body density for a 42-year-old female with a triceps skinfold of 22 mm, suprailium skinfold of 34 mm, and a thigh skinfold of 27 mm.

Step 1: Choose the appropriate equation.

Body density = 1.0994921 − 0.0009929 (Σ3) + 0.0000023 (Σ3)^2 − 0.0001392 (age)

Step 2: Sum the three skinfold sites.

Σ3 = 22 + 34 + 27 = 83

Step 3: Calculate body density.

Body density = 1.0994921 − 0.0009929 (83) + 0.0000023 (83)^2 − 0.0001392 (42)
= 1.02708

The second step in measuring body composition with the skinfold method is calculating percent body fat from body density. Although there are many available equations for calculating percent body fat from body density, the equations developed by Siri (equation 3.7) and Brozek (equation 3.8) are the most common (Brozek, Grande, Anderson, & Keys, 1963; Siri, 1961).

$$\text{Percent body fat} = \left[\left(\frac{4.95}{\text{Body density}}\right) - 4.50\right] \times 100 \tag{3.7}$$

$$\text{Percent body fat} = \left[\left(\frac{4.57}{\text{Body density}}\right) - 4.142\right] \times 100 \tag{3.8}$$

However, despite their widespread use, research has suggested that these equations may not be appropriate when applied to ethnic groups other than whites because of differences in fat-free body density resulting from differences in bone mineral density and body protein content (Wagner & Heyward, 2000). As a result, ethnic-specific equations have been developed for calculating percent body fat from body density, such as Schutte's equation for black males (equation 3.9) (Schutte et al., 1984).

$$\text{Percent body fat} = \left[\left(\frac{4.374}{\text{Body density}}\right) - 3.928\right] \times 100 \tag{3.9}$$

Let's practice calculating percent body from body density using the Siri, Brozec, and Schutte equations.

EXAMPLE 5

Calculate percent body fat for a male with a body density of 1.028 using the Siri, Brozek, and Schutte equations.

1. Siri Equation.

$$\text{Percent body fat} = \left[\frac{4.95}{(1.028)} - 4.50\right] \times 100 = 31.52\%$$

2. Brozek Equation.

$$\text{Percent body fat} = \left[\frac{4.57}{(1.028)} - 4.142\right] \times 100 = 30.35\%$$

3. Schutte Equation.

$$\text{Percent body fat} = \left[\frac{4.374}{(1.028)} - 3.928\right] \times 100 = 32.69\%$$

Measuring Skinfolds in Children and Adolescents   In children and adolescents, percent body fat is calculated directly from skinfold measurements. Slaughter and colleagues developed two sets of sex-specific equations for calculating percent body fat from skinfold measurements in children and adolescents ages 8 through 18 years (Slaughter et al., 1988). Specifically, one set of equations uses the sum of triceps and calf skinfolds, while the other set uses the sum of triceps and subscapular skinfolds. The sex-specific equations for calculating percent body fat from the sum of triceps and calf skinfolds are presented below (equation 3.10 for men and equation 3.11 for women). The nine equations for calculating percent body fat from the sum of triceps and subscapular skinfolds can be found in detail in other sources (Slaughter et al., 1988).

$$\text{Percent body fat} = [0.735 \, (\text{triceps} + \text{calf})] + 1.0 \tag{3.10}$$

$$\text{Percent body fat} = [0.610 \, (\text{triceps} + \text{calf})] + 5.1 \tag{3.11}$$

The three skinfolds are measured at the same location for males and females (Slaughter et al., 1988). The triceps skinfold is a vertical fold that is measured halfway between the olecranon and acromion processes on the posterior upper arm; the subscapula skinfold is measured one centimeter below the inferior angle of the right scapula, inclined downwards and laterally in the natural cleavage of the skin; and the calf skinfold is a vertical fold that is measured on the medial side of the right calf just above the level of maximal calf girth. Let's practice calculating percent body fat from triceps and calf skinfolds.

EXAMPLE 6

Calculate percent body fat for a 13-year-old female with a triceps skinfold of 12 mm and a calf skinfold of 8 mm.

Step 1: Choose the appropriate equation.

Percent body fat = [0.610 (triceps + calf)] + 5.1

Step 2: Calculate percent body fat.

Percent body fat = [0.610 (12 + 8)] + 5.1 = 17.3%

Finally, a single skinfold measurement can be also used to determine whether a child or adolescent has excess body fat. Barlow and Dietz determined that a triceps skinfold thickness greater than the 95th age- and sex-specific percentile is an indicator of excess body fat (Barlow & Dietz, 1998). This approach may be helpful for those using BMI who want to determine whether a child or adolescent has an excessive amount of body fat.

Strengths and Limitations of the Skinfold Method   Although the equipment needed to measure skinfold thickness may cost as much as $400, the cost is significantly less than that of other methods. For example, BIA (bioelectrical impedance analysis) equipment may cost as much as $1,500, and a DXA scanner may cost well over $100,000. In addition, while percent body fat cannot be calculated at specific locations, skinfold thickness at specific locations can be monitored, providing valuable information on regional body composition.

One limitation of the skinfold method is that it can intrude considerably on participant privacy. For example, participants often have to remove some of their clothing so that certain sites can be measured accurately, such as the chest and subscapula sites in men. This can be problematic, particularly when working with children and adolescents, or persons of the sex opposite that of the evaluator. In addition, a considerable amount of training and knowledge of anatomy is required in order to accurately measure skinfold thickness. Finally, this method can difficult to conduct in obese populations since it may difficult to compress their adipose tissue into a fold.

Bioelectrical Impedance Analysis

Bioelectrical impedance analysis (BIA) is a fast, noninvasive, and fairly inexpensive method for measuring body composition. BIA, which involves passing a small electric current through the body and measuring the impedance to that current (Kaminsky, 2006), is an accurate method of measuring body composition in children and adults (Houtkooper, Lohman, Going, & Howell, 1996; Okasora et al., 1999; Tyrrell et al., 2001). For example, Houtkooper and colleagues found that the prediction error of BIA ranged from 1.7 to 3.0 kg for fat-free mass and 0.23 to 1.5 kg for total body water in adults (Houtkooper et al., 1996). In addition, Tyrrell and colleagues found that the body fat determined by BIA was highly correlated, $r = 0.94$, with that of DXA in children (Tyrrell et al., 2001). Although several BIA instruments are available, the hand-to-hand and foot-to-foot instruments are the most commonly used instruments in community and public health settings because they require little training, take little time to use, and place little burden on participants.

The strengths of BIA are that it is a noninvasive, fast, easy-to-use, and accurate method of measuring body composition. BIA is preferred over other methods because it intrudes less on participant privacy. For example, the skinfold method requires participants to remove some of their clothing and to be pinched by an assessor, and the underwater weighing method requires participants to wear a swim suit and be submerged underwater. On the other hand, depending on the instrument used, BIA requires that participants grip a device, remove their shoes and socks, and either stand on a scale or have electrodes placed on their hands and feet. In addition, whereas the skinfold method, underwater weighing, and DXA require a high amount of training, BIA requires little training, particularly when using the hand-to-hand and foot-to-foot devices for which only basic demographic information is entered into the BIA device.

However, BIA does have its limitations. BIA equipment can be expensive: Foot-to-foot analyzers cost as much as $1,500. While the costs associated with BIA are more than those of BMI, waist circumference, and the skinfold method, BIA is significantly less expensive than underwater weighing and DXA. A second limitation is that BIA requires participants to adhere to a number of preparatory guidelines to avoid biasing results, which may be a challenge for participants (Heyward & Wagner, 2004).

Laboratory Methods

This next section focuses on underwater weighing and dual-energy X-ray absorptiometry (DXA). As previously mentioned, the focus of this chapter is on field methods. As a result, underwater weighing and DXA are not discussed in as much detail as the field methods already discussed. It should also be noted that, although it is not discussed in this chapter, the Bod Pod is another commonly used laboratory method for measuring body composition.

Underwater Weighing

The purpose of underwater weighing is to measure body volume, which is then used to calculate body density, followed by the percent body fat calculation. Although no longer considered the gold standard of body composition measurements, underwater weighing is an extremely accurate method and is still used in many laboratories and settings. In terms of accuracy, the standard error associated with underwater weighing is about 2.5% body fat (Nash, 1985); the largest source of error involves the measurement of residual lung volume (Baumgartner et al., 2003). Specifically, each 100 ml error in lung volume results in a .7% error in percent body fat (Baumgartner et al., 2003). As a result, it's recommended that residual volume be measured rather than estimated in order to obtain the most accurate measurement possible.

Although extremely accurate, underwater weighing does have limitations. First, underwater weighing requires the use of expensive equipment, such as a water tank, harnesses, and suspension equipment, a force transducer or scale, equipment to measure residual volume, and tank cleaning supplies. Second, this method is invasive; participants are required to submerge themselves underwater for up to fifteen seconds for five to twelve trials (Adams, 2002). This can be problematic for those who are uncomfortable being underwater and for populations such as children, the elderly, and individuals with disabilities. In addition, underwater weighing requires a considerable amount of time to conduct and typically requires participants to visit a laboratory, which can place a large burden on participants. Finally, because participants are submerging themselves underwater, test administrators should be certified in first aid and CPR and must be able to judge when a correct trial has taken place. As a result, assessors must complete a considerable amount of training.

> How might a researcher or community practitioner decide which body composition assessment to use?

Dual-Energy X-ray Absorptiometry

Dual-energy X-ray absorptiometry (DXA) is one of the most common laboratory methods for measuring body composition and has replaced underwater weighing as the gold standard for measuring body composition. DXA measures body composition by using X-rays to segment the body into three components—fat mass, bone-free lean tissue, and bone mineral mass—and has the ability to provide total and regional percent body fat. In addition to providing information on percent body fat, DXA is a common diagnostic tool for osteoporosis.

Although DXA is extremely accurate, can provide information on regional body composition, and is a diagnostic tool for osteoporosis, it does have its limitations. Perhaps most important, a DXA scanner can cost well over $100,000, and the cost of a single scan can exceed $100 at a laboratory. The body size the DXA scanner can assess is also limited. A person cannot be too wide or too large, anterior to posterior: The arm of the DXA scanner is limited in height and the width of the area measured by the DXA machine is limited as well. As a result, it may not be possible to use this method with severely obese individuals.

GETTING STARTED

❏ Determine your purpose for measuring body composition.

❏ Determine what monetary and personal resources are available.

❏ Consider the population you will be working with.

❏ Consider the burden your chosen method will place on participants.

❏ Plan on how to assist and intervene with overweight and obese individuals.

❏ Practice your chosen method of body composition assessment repeatedly.

Summary

Although they are less accurate than laboratory methods, field methods are commonly used in community and public health settings because of the lower cost associated with them and the low burden they place on participants. Determining which method is most appropriate for one's needs is an important step, whether or not the purpose is for research. As a result, the information presented in this chapter should be taken into careful consideration when deciding which method is most appropriate for one's purpose and population.

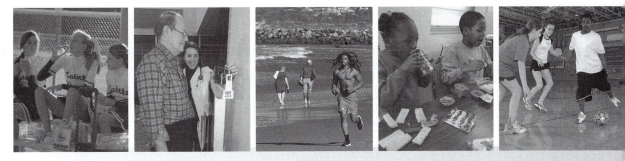

Physical Activity and Obesity

The second part of this book is related primarily to environmental factors that foster physical activity. Physical activity plays an important part in healthy weight maintenance. And as described in the U.S. National Physical Activity Plan (2010), environments that foster physical activity are vital if we expect people to be physically active. The research literature shows a clear relationship between features of the built environment, access to physical activity resources, and active transportation systems and regular physical activity. This part of the text describes these relationships and discusses strategies for defining and documenting neighborhood factors important for enhancing physical activity. These factors are often driven by policy and community considerations, and so there are connections between this part and other parts of the book that consider policy and community factors. As well, the human-developed cities that include the built environment, physical activity resources, and transportation systems contribute to the food environment, so there is some affinity between this part and those that address food access and policy.

PART

two

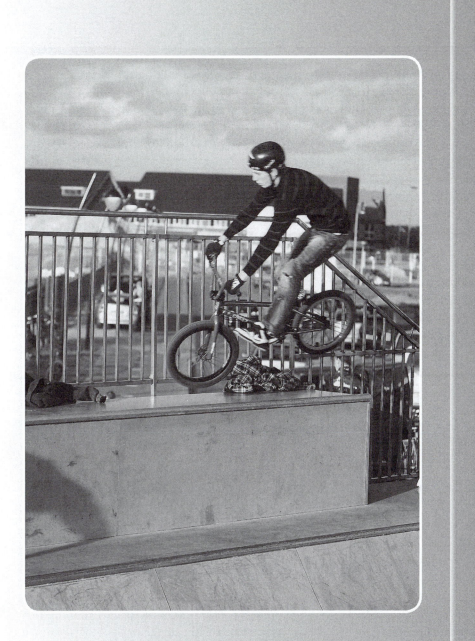

CHAPTER 4

The Built Environment

Despite efforts by public health professionals, researchers, and policy professionals to promote physical activity and to prevent overweight and obesity, observational data indicate that little progress has been made in these efforts (CDC, 2007; Flegal, Carroll, Ogden, & Curtin, 2010; Ogden, Carroll, Curtin, Lamb, & Flegal, 2010; Troiano et al., 2008). Researchers in a variety of disciplines have moved away from a paradigm that focused almost entirely on individual characteristics toward one that incorporates the social and built environments in which people live and interact. Research examining the influence of the built environment on individual health behaviors, which has primarily grown out of transportation literature linking it to physical activity, is one promising area that has emerged from this paradigm shift.

This chapter provides an introduction to the built environment by exploring various aspects of its relationship with physical activity and obesity. This chapter defines the built environment and its components, discusses methods of measuring the built environment for physical activity, examines the built environment's relationship with physical activity and obesity, and provides recommendations for public health practitioners, researchers, policy professionals, and the general public.

Components of the Built Environment

The built environment refers to the physical form of a neighborhood, community, or city and includes the roads, buildings, food sources, and recreation facilities available to its residents for shopping, working, and playing (Frank, Engelke, & Schmidt, 2003; Sallis & Glanz, 2006). Components of the built environment can be divided into neighborhood or regional scales (Handy, Boarnet, Ewing, & Killingsworth, 2002). Because neighborhood characteristics are likely to have a greater influence on individual health

---

Built + environment = the human-made physical form of a neighborhood, community, or city.

---

behaviors, such as physical activity and healthful eating, and potentially have a stronger relationship with overweight and obesity, only neighborhood-scale components are discussed. These include density and intensity, land-use mix, street connectivity, street scale, and aesthetic quality.

Density and intensity refer to the amount of activity that takes place within an area, based on the number of people, households, or jobs (Frumkin, Frank, & Jackson, 2004; Handy et al., 2002). This can be measured as the population or number of jobs within a square mile or kilometer, census tract, or any other boundary (Frumkin et al., 2004). Let's use the cities of Houston and Philadelphia as examples of population density. Houston has a greater population than Philadelphia; however, Philadelphia has a greater population density. This is because Philadelphia has a much smaller geographic space for people to live when compared to Houston. Although there are fewer people living in

Philadelphia, because they live in a smaller geographic space, Philadelphia is a denser city (Gibson, 1998).

Land-use mix refers to the various types of land uses that are within an area, such as residential housing, business offices, entertainment facilities, stores, restaurants, parks, and recreational facilities (Frumkin et al., 2004; Handy et al., 2002). New York City is an example of an area with a diverse land-use mix because residences, businesses, and recreational opportunities are located near one another. On the other hand, suburban and rural areas are often recognized as having little land-use mix because residences, businesses, and recreational opportunities are usually located far from one another.

Street connectivity refers to how travel destinations are linked in transportation systems and serves as an indicator of the directness and availability of routes within a street network (Frumkin et al., 2004; Handy et al., 2002). Street connectivity is often measured by the number of intersections within a given area, or the ratio between the straight line distance and the distance along the street network between two points (Handy et al., 2002). Urban areas typically have a higher street connectivity than suburban and rural areas, primarily because of their gridlike nature. Suburban and rural areas tend to have a higher number of dead ends, cul-de-sacs, and long streets; as a result, they typically have lower street connectivity.

Street scale refers to the space along a street whose boundary is set by buildings; it can be measured by the ratio of building heights to street widths or by the average distance from the street to the buildings (Handy et al., 2002). Building height and street width are important factors for street segment use, particularly for pedestrian use (e.g., sidewalks, bike lanes). For example, taller buildings can provide more segment enclosure and shade for pedestrians, wider sidewalks and public spaces can provide more space for walking and other forms of physical activity, and bike lanes can offer a safe place for bicyclists to ride.

Aesthetic quality refers to the attractiveness or appeal of a place. It can include characteristics such as building design, cleanliness and maintenance, and the presence of trees and shade (Frumkin et al., 2004; Handy et al., 2002). Aesthetic qualities are important features of the built environment and have been shown to be associated with various health behaviors and outcomes. For example, the aesthetic qualities of physical activity resources are associated with increased physical activity and lower body mass index among community residents (Heinrich et al., 2008; Heinrich et al., 2007).

Measuring the Built Environment

There are various ways to measure the built environment and its suitability for physical activity and for categorizing these measurement methods. For the purpose of this chapter, methods of measuring the built environment are divided into three categories: self-report methods, geographic information systems-based measures (GIS-based measures), and observational assessment methods (Brownson, Hoehner, Day, Forsyth, & Sallis, 2009). Methods of measuring the food environment are not discussed; however, information on this subject can be found in a review by McKinnon and colleagues (McKinnon, Reedy, Morrissette, Lytle, & Yaroch, 2009).

Self-Report Methods

Self-report methods of measuring the built environment involve the use of surveys to obtain people's perceptions of their environment. Several surveys have been developed, ranging considerably in the environmental attributes they assess and in their comprehensiveness. A review by Brownson and colleagues identified 15 adult surveys and 4 child and adolescent surveys, with survey length ranging from 7 to 68 items (Brownson et al., 2009). When choosing the most appropriate survey for one's needs, it's important to select a survey that has adequate reliability and validity, assesses the environmental attributes of interest, and was developed in populations (e.g., children) and geographic regions (e.g., urban environments) similar to those that will be assessed.

The Neighborhood Environment Walkability Scale (NEWS) (figure 4.1) is an example of a self-report survey used to measure people's perceptions of their environment (Saelens, Sallis, Black, & Chen, 2003). The NEWS instrument contains 68 items; there is also an abbreviated 54-item version (ANEWS) (Cerin, Saelens, Sallis, & Frank, 2006). This survey is a great example of a simple way to obtain information on residential density, land use, street connectivity, walking and cycling facilities, aesthetics, pedestrian and traffic safety, and crime safety. The NEWS and ANEWS instruments have been used in a variety of populations and display adequate test-retest reliability (Cerin et al., 2006; Saelens et al., 2003).

Self-report surveys have several strengths over GIS-based measures and observational assessment methods. Self-report surveys are less time consuming, because it may take only 5 to 15 minutes per participant to complete a survey. On the other hand, depending on the protocol used, collecting environment data using observational assessment methods may take many hours, days, or weeks to assess a single neighborhood or community. In addition, the only costs associated with self-report surveys are those associated with photocopying the survey and entering survey responses into a database. This is a considerable strength, because GIS-based measures and observational assessment methods have high costs associated with their use. Last, self-report surveys don't require the use of well-trained auditors, GIS experts, or individuals with any particular expertise.

However, self-report surveys do have their limitations. Perhaps the greatest limitation of self-report surveys is bias on the participant's part, such as not answering specific items, incorrectly identifying available goods and services in their community, and inappropriately describing environmental conditions, such as safety and sidewalk conditions. In addition, self-report surveys may suffer from low return and high refusal rates.

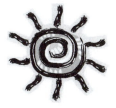

Neighborhood Environment Walkability Scale (NEWS)

We would like to find out more information about the way that you perceive or think about your neighborhood. Please answer the following questions about your neighborhood and yourself. Please answer as honestly and completely as possible and provide only one answer for each item. There are no right or wrong answers and your information is kept confidential.

A. Types of residences in your neighborhood

Among the residences in your neighborhood...

	None	A few	Some	Most	All
1. How common are detached single-family residences in your immediate neighborhood?	O	O	O	O	O
2. How common are townhouses or row houses of 1-3 stories in your immediate neighborhood?	O	O	O	O	O
3. How common are apartments or condos 1-3 stories in your immediate neighborhood?	O	O	O	O	O
4. How common are apartments or condos 4-6 stories in your immediate neighborhood?	O	O	O	O	O
5. How common are apartments or condos 7-12 stories in your immediate neighborhood?	O	O	O	O	O
6. How common are apartments or condos more than 13 stories in your immediate neighborhood?	O	O	O	O	O

FIGURE 4.1 Section A of the NEWS instrument.

Adapted, by permission, from B.E. Saelens and J.F. Sallis, 2002, Neighborhood Environment Walkability Survey. [Online]. Available: www.activelivingresearch.org/node/10649 [November 1, 2010].

Geographic Information Systems-Based Measures

Geographic information systems (GIS) are the integration of hardware, software, and data for capturing, managing, analyzing, and displaying all forms of geographically referenced information (ESRI, 2010) and is an important tool used by public health practitioners and researchers. GIS can be used in many ways relative to physical activity and obesity. For example, GIS can be used to create maps that can be used for observational assessment data collection purposes (figure 4.2), to display data, such the location of physical activity resources across a region by socioeconomic status, or to calculate variables that can be used for data analysis purposes.

Although an in-depth description of GIS-based measures is beyond the scope of this chapter, some of the more commonly assessed measures related to physical activity and obesity include population density, land-use mix, access to recreational facilities, street patterns, sidewalk coverage, traffic and crime safety, and various indices and composite scores (Brownson et al., 2009). Data used for GIS purposes are usually obtained from the U.S. census data and from local city and government agencies. In addition, many commercial businesses have GIS data available for purchase; however, these can be quite expensive.

GIS has many strengths. The greatest strength is that it is the only feasible method for obtaining objective environment data in projects involving a large number of individuals or individuals from several geographic regions. For example, it may not be feasible to use observational assessment methods in a study that involves hundreds or thousands of participants or in a study where participants are located in multiple cities or states. In addition, recall biases, which are a concern with self-report methods, are not applicable to

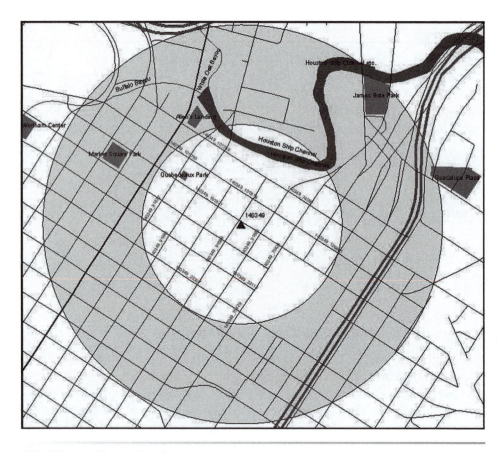

FIGURE 4.2   Observational assessment map.

GIS-based measures. Finally, while obtaining data and securing staff trained in GIS can be expensive, the cost associated with using GIS-based measures may be less than conducting observational assessment methods.

Although they can be a powerful tool in public health research, GIS-based measures do have their limitations. Knowing how to obtain, use, and analyze GIS data requires trained personnel and sufficient time to do the training. In addition, while some GIS data can be obtained for free, commercially obtained data can be quite expensive. Similarly, the software needed to work with GIS data can be quite expensive. An additional limitation is that, whether free or purchased, the data may contain inaccuracies that could lead to biased associations. Little research evidence is available concerning the accuracy of GIS data. Because GIS data are not typically collected with a specific research purpose in mind, there are often inconsistencies and irregularities. In the work of the authors and others, we have observed many inconsistencies between what we have measured during observational assessments and what GIS data reported to have existed. Last, the nature and scope of available GIS data and the methodologies used to collect and aggregate them can vary widely from one municipality to the next, making comparisons across municipalities challenging.

Observational Assessment Methods

Observational assessment methods to measure the built environment involve trained staff going into neighborhoods and communities to perform in-person audits of the environment. The specific factors that are measured depend on the audit instrument that is used, but at minimum usually include an assessment of pedestrian and bicycling environments. Some of the more commonly assessed factors include residential housing, street conditions, sidewalk conditions, aesthetic qualities, traffic and crime safety, nonresidential land use (e.g., grocery stores, restaurants, churches), and the availability and quality of physical activity resources.

In-person audits can be conducted by a single person or by a team of auditors. Data collection with a team of auditors is preferred because it affords greater safety, offers opportunities to examine interrater reliability, and is often more enjoyable. Field auditors receive a considerable amount of training before data collection to ensure they understand the nature and scope of the data collection instruments.

Training usually involves a classroom-based learning component during which field auditors are given background information on the purpose of the project and detailed information on data collection protocols and instrument operational definitions. After this classroom-based learning experience, trainees may practice by assessing environments that are similar to those they will assess under the supervision of their trainers. This practice may then be followed by shadowing experienced auditors during real data collection, allowing them to ask questions and verify data collection procedures. This shadowing experience allows trainees to observe and experience data collection in a safe and productive manner. Trainees should train until they have demonstrated a high amount of agreement with their trainers. In addition, interrater reliability should be monitored throughout data collection.

Several instruments are available for assessing the built environment for physical activity, each developed for a specific environment (e.g., urban, rural). Four of the most common instruments are the Systematic Pedestrian and Cycling Environmental Scan (SPACES) (Pikora et al., 2002), the Irvine Minnesota Inventory (Boarnet, Day, Alfonzo, Forsyth, & Oakes, 2006), the Analytic Audit Tool and Checklist Audit Tool (Brownson, 2004), and the Pedestrian Environment Data Scan (PEDS) Tool (Clifton, Livi Smith, & Rodriguez, 2007). These instruments have displayed adequate reliability and vary in terms of the components of the built environment they assess. Although many instruments are available for conducting in-person audits, this chapter discusses only the PEDS (Clifton et al., 2007) and Goods and Services Inventory (GASI) instruments (Lee, Liao, & McAlexander, 2009).

Pedestrian Environment Data Scan (PEDS) Tool   The PEDS tool is used by trained auditors to assess individual street segments (Clifton et al., 2007), which are portions of a street that are intersected by two cross streets or by a cross street at one end and a dead end or cul-de-sac at the other. The PEDS tool contains 40 items and assesses components of the built environment such as residential and nonresidential land use, pedestrian facilities, road attributes, walking and cycling environments, safety, and aesthetics. To assess individual street segments, audit teams carry a map of the area they are going to assess with identified street segments (see figure 4.2 on page 52). Using this map, team members assess each street segment with the audit instrument, completing one PEDS for every street segment.

Goods and Services Inventory (GASI)   The Goods and Services Inventory (GASI) is an audit instrument that can be used to record the number of nonresidential land uses on a street segment, specifically places that can be used to obtain goods and services (figure 4.3). These include table service, fast food, and other types of restaurants; supermarkets, grocery stores, pharmacies, and gas station and convenience stores; banks, credit unions, pawn shops, and check cashing stores; liquor stores, tobacco stores, bars, and nightclubs; adult video stores and sex-related businesses; places of worship; salons, barbers, and beauty shops; schools and day care facilities; and libraries. As with the PEDS tool, audit teams carry a map of the area they are going to assess with street segments indicated for assessment. Using this map, team members assess each indicated street segment with the audit instrument, completing one GASI for every street segment.

Choosing the instrument that is most appropriate for one's needs can be a difficult task. Although the majority of audit instruments are comprehensive in their assessment of the built environment, they don't assess every aspect of the built environment. Auditors have to determine which instrument is

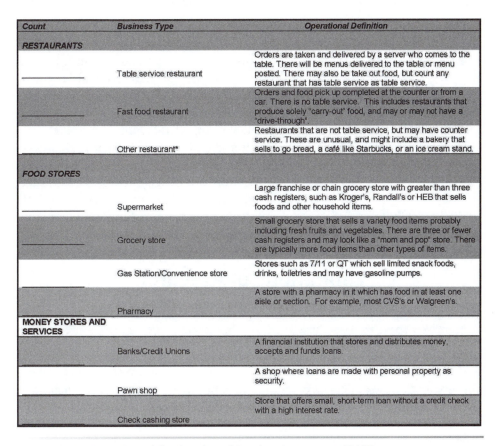

Count	Business Type	Operational Definition
RESTAURANTS		
	Table service restaurant	Orders are taken and delivered by a server who comes to the table. There will be menus delivered to the table or menu posted. There may also be take out food, but count any restaurant that has table service as table service.
	Fast food restaurant	Orders and food pick up completed at the counter or from a car. There is no table service. This includes restaurants that produce solely "carry-out" food, and may or may not have a "drive-through".
	Other restaurant*	Restaurants that are not table service, but may have counter service. These are unusual, and might include a bakery that sells to go bread, a café like Starbucks, or an ice cream stand.
FOOD STORES		
	Supermarket	Large franchise or chain grocery store with greater than three cash registers, such as Kroger's, Randall's or HEB that sells foods and other household items.
	Grocery store	Small grocery store that sells a variety food items probably including fresh fruits and vegetables. There are three or fewer cash registers and may look like a "mom and pop" store. There are typically more food items than other types of items.
	Gas Station/Convenience store	Stores such as 7/11 or QT which sell limited snack foods, drinks, toiletries and may have gasoline pumps.
	Pharmacy	A store with a pharmacy in it which has food in at least one aisle or section. For example, most CVS's or Walgreen's.
MONEY STORES AND SERVICES		
	Banks/Credit Unions	A financial institution that stores and distributes money, accepts and funds loans.
	Pawn shop	A shop where loans are made with personal property as security.
	Check cashing store	Store that offers small, short-term loan without a credit check with a high interest rate.

FIGURE 4.3   A portion of the Goods and Services Instrument (GASI).

Used with permission of Rebecca Lee.

most appropriate and comprehensive for their purpose; often this results in researchers selecting multiple instruments or adapting existing instruments. For example, if auditors were interested in comprehensively assessing nonresidential land use and pedestrian and cycling environments, they may use the PEDS and GASI to obtain a comprehensive assessment of the environment.

The primary strength of the observational assessment methods is that environments are measured based on what is present in the environment. Rather than rely on residents' perceptions or on databases that may be inaccurate or outdated, trained auditors go into the field to accurately record the presence and quality of various environmental variables. However, this objectivity comes at a high cost. Perhaps the greatest limitation of observational assessment methods is that they are time consuming and expensive to conduct, particularly when several neighborhoods and communities must be assessed. For example, it takes an average of 5 to 10 minutes to assess one segment using the PEDS tool and an average of 10 to 20 minutes using the Irvine Minnesota Inventory and the Analytic Audit Tool and Checklist Audit Tool. In neighborhoods with a high street-segment density, a full sample of street segments within a half-mile radius of a selected address can equate to hundreds of street segments and several days or weeks of data collection per neighborhood. Even in areas with a lower street-segment density, data collection time and cost are significant. As a result, abbreviated data collection protocols using systematic street segment sampling protocols have been developed (McMillan, Cubbin, Parmenter, Medina, & Lee, 2010). However, even when using these abbreviated data collection protocols, the costs associated with data collection can be substantial if a large number of neighborhoods must be assessed.

What do you think are stronger predictors of physical activity: residents' perceptions of their neighborhood, or what is present in their neighborhood? How do you think this question shapes research on the built environment and physical activity promotion efforts?

Limitations of Research on the Built Environment

Now that we have discussed individual components of the built environment and methods for measuring the built environment for physical activity, we can discuss possible ways that the built environment influences physical activity and obesity. This next section does not focus on specific associations because there are several literature reviews on the topic (Casagrande, Whitt-Glover, Lancaster, Odoms-Young, & Gary, 2009; Duncan, Spence, & Mummery, 2005; Dunton, Kaplan, Wolch, Jerrett, & Reynolds, 2009; Feng, Glass, Curriero, Stewart, & Schwartz, 2010; Owen, Humpel, Leslie, Bauman, & Sallis, 2004; Papas et al., 2007; Sallis & Glanz, 2006; Wendel-Vos, Droomers, Kremers, Brug, & van Lenthe, 2007), but instead discusses limitations in the existing research literature.

The greatest limitation in the literature on built environment is that a majority of the research to date has been conducted using cross-sectional study designs. In cross-sectional designs, information on one's environment, individual health behavior (e.g., physical activity), and health are collected at the same time. This prevents researchers from making causal inferences concerning the built environment. Research studies using longitudinal study designs have begun to be published more often; however, there are several methodological concerns with these studies, and the body of literature to date is quite small. Although research has provided evidence for a relationship between the built environment and physical activity and obesity, we do not know if physical activity-friendly environments make neighborhood residents more physically active and less obese, if active and fit residents seek out or create environments supportive of physical activity, or if some other variable or combination of variables influences both.

Measurement is another limitation in the research on built environment. A considerable number of technological advances have been made in the area of

GIS-based measures over the past few years, and several self-report surveys and observational assessment instruments have been developed as well. Although these advances further the field of research on the built environment, there are many concerns surrounding their use. For example, there is currently no consensus regarding how to calculate GIS-based measures, and unfortunately few researchers in the past have provided enough detail in their manuscripts to allow others to calculate variables in a similar manner (Brownson et al., 2009). In addition, there is no consensus concerning how to best aggregate or present data collected from observational assessment instruments. As a result, researchers often create indices using different methods yet call their variables by the same name (e.g., walkability).

These measurement issues are compounded by the fact that a majority of research studies to date have relied on self-report measures of physical activity and the built environment. This is in part due to the laborious nature of observational assessment methods and GIS-based measures and uncertainties about how to best handle and analyze these data. As a result of these measurement issues, it's not surprising that researchers have found inconsistent results and that the associations found thus far have been weak (Dunton et al., 2009; Wendel-Vos et al., 2007).

Although the research literature has produced inconsistent results, some aspects of the built environment have consistently been associated with physical activity, leading to intervention and policy efforts aimed at increasing physical activity and reducing obesity. The following section focuses on one such aspect of the built environment, walkability, and current initiatives to make communities more walkable.

Neighborhood Walkability and Physical Activity

Walkability is a variable composed of several aspects of the built environment (e.g., street connectivity, land-use mix) that was developed to describe the supportiveness of neighborhoods and communities for walking and being physically active. Although the effects have been small, the research literature has consistently shown that walkable communities are associated with increased physical activity among neighborhood residents. Adults living in highly walkable neighborhoods do more moderate- and vigorous-intensity physical activity (Sallis et al., 2009), are more likely to meet physical activity recommendations (Frank, Schmid, Sallis, Chapman, & Saelens, 2005), and are less likely to be overweight and obese (Frank, Andresen, & Schmid, 2004; Sallis et al., 2009) when compared to adults living in low walkable neighborhoods.

Similar results have been found when examining similar aspects of the built environment. For example, neighborhoods with sidewalks that are shaded, well maintained, and well lit with streetlights tend to have residents who are more physically active (Frank et al., 2005; Jago, Baranowski, Baranowski,

Thompson, & Greaves, 2005; Reed, Wilson, Ainsworth, Bowles, & Mixon, 2006). In addition, several research studies have found that people living in areas with high population density, greater street connectivity, and greater access to goods and services tend to have residents who weigh less (Lavizzo-Mourey, 2008). As a result of these and other findings, public health professionals, community planners, and policy professionals have begun calling for legislation to make neighborhoods more walkable. They've had some success with the passing of legislation to improve the land-use mix of neighborhoods throughout California (Office of the Governor, 2008), and with the passing of complete street acts in several states (National Complete Streets Coalition, n.d.).

Although they are usually not components of walkability indices, neighborhood aesthetics and safety are factors that can strongly influence whether people are physically active, and they deserve comment in this chapter. Research has shown that adolescents who perceived their neighborhood as more aesthetically pleasing were more physically active than those who perceived poorer quality neighborhoods (Mota, Almeida, Santos, & Ribeiro, 2005). Parental concerns about safety are also important because the parents may prevent children from being physically active; these parental concerns have been associated with greater overweight among children (Dwyer et al., 2006; Lumeng, Appugliese, Cabral, Bradley, & Zuckerman, 2006). Similarly, adolescent girls and women have reported that they avoided using physical activity resources because they perceived them as being unsafe (Dwyer et al., 2006; Gomez, Johnson, Selva, & Sallis, 2004). It isn't clear whether perceived

Implementing Policy

Complete Street Acts

Efforts to make communities more supportive of physical activity have primarily focused on passing legislation known as complete street acts. Complete street acts are legislation developed to ensure that all users of transportation systems (including pedestrians, bicyclists, transit users, individuals with disabilities, and individuals of all ages) are able to travel safely and conveniently on all federally funded streets and highways. This type of legislation has passed in communities throughout the United States (National Complete Streets Coalition, n.d.). In addition, a complete streets act was introduced to the U.S. Congress in 2009 and is currently under review by the Committee on Environment and Public Works (S. 584: Complete Streets Act of 2009, 2010). Although these efforts are promising, making widespread changes to communities and existing infrastructures may take a considerable amount of time to accomplish. Thus, in addition to pursuing these efforts, it's important to also focus on smaller efforts within individual communities, many of which can be undertaken by community residents and public health practitioners.

safety corresponds to actual safety. However, research has shown that neighborhoods that have a considerable amount of social disorder (e.g., graffiti, public intoxication, litter, broken windows, abandoned cars) have residents who feel less safe and who are less physically active (Molnar, Gortmaker, Bull, & Buka, 2004; Sampson & Raudenbush, 2004).

In addition to its relationship to physical activity, urban form can also be related to the distribution of food sources, which in turn may affect dietary habits and ultimately overweight and obesity. For example, research has indicated that urban neighborhoods are more likely to have convenience stores, small grocery stores, and liquor stores rather than large commercial supermarkets (Lee et al., 2009; Sooman, Macintyre, & Anderson, 1993). This has important implications: Neighborhood residents who rely on these stores for their food often have a limited selection of healthful foods,

> What is the nature and extent of the role that the built environment plays in physical activity and obesity?

which are also available at higher costs (Sooman et al., 1993). Similarly, low socioeconomic status neighborhoods may lack healthful eating options, have fewer supermarkets, and have higher costs for those options that are available (Morland, Wing, Diez Roux, & Poole, 2002). This is also important since research has shown that living near a supermarket is associated with eating more fruits and vegetables and consuming less fat (Morland, Wing, & Diez Roux, 2002). Information about retail food outlets is discussed in detail in chapter 13.

Emerging Research and Recommendations

Although the cross-sectional studies conducted to date have been extremely valuable, it's important that the field begin addressing some research issues. First, researchers must use longitudinal study designs more regularly. The use of longitudinal designs provides stronger evidence for causal relationships and additional support for changing environments in an effort to promote physical activity and to prevent obesity. Second, it is important that researchers begin standardizing data collection protocols, GIS-based measures, and the aggregation of data obtained from observational assessment methods. Finally, it is important that as natural changes to environments take place (e.g., passage of complete streets acts, changes in land use), those changes be evaluated in terms of whether community residents engage in more physical activity. This can provide information for optimizing future physical activity promotion efforts.

Last, it's important that researchers, practitioners, policy makers, and community members all begin to move forward with efforts to create environments that promote physical activity and healthful dietary habits. Although there are limitations in the existing research literature, several associations have consistently been found. In addition, it intuitively makes sense that having a safe environment that encourages physical activity will aide in promoting physical activity. Some communities have begun to move forward with such efforts; however, greater resources in terms of political will, grassroots support, and funding are needed (CDC, 2008; "Strategic Alliance Newsletter," 2008).

GETTING STARTED

❏ Determine the specific components of the built environment that are most important for answering the question under investigation.

❏ Determine whether GIS-based measures and observational assessment methods are necessary, or if self-report methods can be used.

❏ Identify potential sources of funding to make your community more supportive of physical activity.

❏ Develop a plan to sustain environmental changes that accommodates the community and citizens.

Summary

Despite limitations in the research literature, when all of the available information is taken into account, the built environment is shown to influence physical activity and ultimately overweight and obesity. Combined with individually based promotion efforts, efforts to create environments that are supportive of physical activity hold promise for promoting physical activity and decreasing the prevalence of overweight and obesity among all populations. Efforts need to be taken to create environments supportive of physical activity and their effectiveness needs to be examined in terms of their use, sustainability, and impact on the physical activity habits and weight status of community residents.

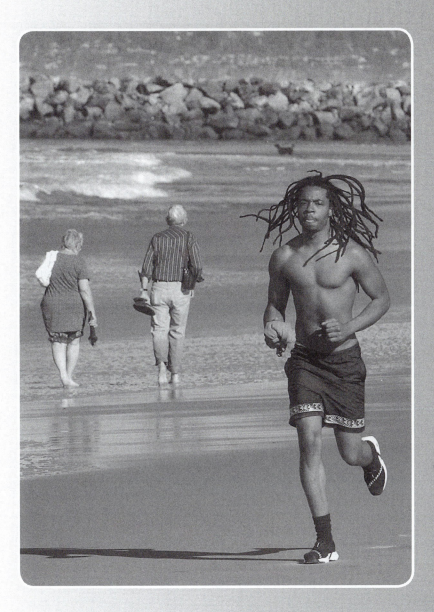

CHAPTER 5

Physical Activity Resources

The research literature on the built environment has consistently shown that physical activity resources are an important factor in promoting physical activity and, as a result, are beginning to play a more prominent role in efforts to create environments supportive of physical activity. Physical activity resources refer to any public or private setting, facility, equipment, or program that promotes and fosters physical activity. Ideally, these resources should be free of charge but can include places that are also fee based. Free resources include parks, open spaces, walking trails, bikeways, and other publicly available resources that do not require a fee, dues, or a paid membership. Fee-based resources are resources that require a fee, dues, or a paid membership to use, such as gyms, recreational centers, swimming pools, dance studios, golf courses, and sport organizations.

As industrialized nations continue to move toward a more technologically advanced, sedentary society, it is important to identify which physical activity resources are available in communities and which specific factors contribute to their use in order to more effectively promote physical activity and reduce the prevalence of obesity. To understand how physical activity resources are perceived and used by community residents, several instruments have been developed that allow researchers to assess the positive and negative aspects of physical activity resources. These instruments can be used in measuring the attributes of physical activity resources, including features, amenities, and incivilities.

This chapter highlights the importance of physical activity resources, their relationship to physical activity, methods for assessing physical activity resources, and efforts to renovate and build physical activity resources in communities. Because many physical activity resources are available across various types of settings, discussing the full spectrum of resources in depth is beyond the scope of this chapter. As a result, this chapter primarily focuses on parks, open spaces, walking trails, and bikeways, because they are the most common resources available in communities and because they have been the primary focus of research studies and efforts to create environments conducive to physical activity. This next section begins by discussing various types of physical activity resources, including parks, open spaces, and other common resources.

Parks and Open Spaces

Within the expanded paradigm discussed in chapter 4, parks and open spaces have been identified as an important setting for physical activity. Parks and open spaces are community features that provide an ideal setting for physical activity because they offer a free or low-cost alternative to other resources, making them accessible to most people. For example, Bedimo-Rung and colleagues illustrated in their conceptual model that parks can play an important role in helping individuals and communities reach public health recommendations for physical activity by providing places to be physically active (Bedimo-Rung, Mowen, & Cohen, 2005). In addition, parks and open spaces are particularly important since they are capable of accommodating many people and uses at the same time.

In addition to providing individual benefits, parks and open spaces have the potential to positively affect communities. On a community level, parks and open spaces facilitate community interactions by providing a common meeting place for people, thereby increasing community cohesion, the strong and positive relationships that are developed within a community by its residents. Social capital, the social networks and interactions that inspire trust and reciprocity among community residents, is also greater in communities with parks and open spaces (Cohen, et al., 2008). In addition to these social benefits, communities can benefit economically from parks and open spaces. For example, residential and commercial property values are typically higher when in proximity to parks and open spaces (Crompton, 2005). Furthermore, businesses that are close to parks are frequented more often than similar businesses that are not near parks.

On an individual level, research has indicated that having more physical activity resources available can facilitate active forms of transportation, such as walking and bicycling (Zlot & Schmid, 2005). Further, Parks and colleagues found that, as the number of available physical activity resources available to individuals increased, their likelihood of meeting physical activity recommendations also increased (Parks, Housemann, & Brownson, 2003). Parks and open spaces are believed to provide several psychological health benefits as well. For example, users of parks and open spaces have reported reduced stress, anxiety, sadness, and depression, along with improved mood and an overall enhanced sense of wellness (Bedimo-Rung et al., 2005).

Despite these benefits, communities vary considerably in the number of parks they have available: Availability often depends on funding and land use. For example, cities such as San Francisco, San Diego, and Washington, DC, have devoted almost 20% of their acreage to parks and open spaces (Zlot & Schmid, 2005). In comparison, cities such as San Jose and Atlanta have devoted less than 4% of their acreage to parks and open spaces. As a result, communities vary considerably in their exposure to parks and open spaces, and ultimately, in the benefits that they provide as well.

Walking Trails and Bikeways

Walking trails and bikeways are physical activity resources with enormous potential to promote physical activity. Research has indicated that walking is the most common form of physical activity done by Americans, and in many other countries as well (CDC, 2001; WHO, 2009). In the United States, nearly 45% of adults report that they walk as a form of physical activity. Although less prevalent than walkways, bikeways are common features most often

Renovating and Building Physical Activity Resources

Several local, state, and federal agencies, along with various private foundations and nonprofit organizations, have begun efforts to renovate and build physical activity resources in communities throughout the United States. The state of California, for example, passed Assembly Bill 31, which prioritized $400 million of Proposition 84 park funds to underserved and park-poor communities throughout California (Office of the Governor, 2008). In addition, since 2002, the Tony Hawk Foundation has awarded over 450 grants totaling more than $2.6 million to build skate parks in low-income communities (The Tony Hawk Foundation, 2010).

Two prominent nonprofit organizations that have been influential in creating communities supportive of physical activity are the Rails-to-Trails Conservancy and the Trust for Public Land. The Rails-to-Trails Conservancy is a nonprofit organization whose mission is to create a nationwide network of trails from rail lines and connecting corridors to built healthier places for healthier people (Rails-to-Trails Conservancy, 2007). Similarly, the Trust for Public Land is a nonprofit organization that conserves land for people to enjoy as parks, community gardens, historic sites, rural lands, and other natural places. The Trust for Public Land has been extremely productive in their efforts, having assisted states and communities in passing over 380 ballot measures and generating $36 billion in new conservation-related funding since 1994 (The Trust for Public Land, 2010).

found as separate lanes in streets or as specifically designated paths in parks and open spaces. For example, some communities, such as the cities in the San Francisco Bay Area, have designated roadways specifically for bicycling and provide interconnected commuting maps for bicycling enthusiasts (San Francisco Bicycle Coalition, 2009). As a result of their popularity, efforts are in place to create and renovate walking trails and bikeways in various communities throughout the United States.

Home Environment

Home-based physical activity resources are any equipment or opportunity that can be used for physical activity in a home setting; these might include treadmills, stationary bikes, running shoes, a dog, and exercise videos and DVDs. Previous research has shown that people with access to home exercise equipment tend to be more physically active and have lower rates of obesity (Johnson-Down, O'Loughlin, Koski, & Gray-Donald, 1997; Reed & Phillips, 2005; Trost, Pate, Ward, Saunders, & Riner, 1999). Similar results have been seen among high school girls (Trost et al., 1999), college students (Reed & Phillips, 2005; Sallis, Johnson, Calfas, Caparosa, & Nichols, 1997), and adults (Ham & Epping, 2006), where increased access to home exercise equipment was associated with increased physical activity.

Factors Influencing the Use of Physical Activity Resources

Many factors influence whether people use physical activity resources. Discussing all of these factors is not feasible within this chapter. Instead, we discuss the more common factors examined in the research literature, including those we think are the strongest predictors of physical activity resource use: accessibility, proximity, safety, and the presence and quality of features and amenities, aesthetics, and incivilities.

Accessibility

Accessibility is composed of many factors that influence the use of physical activity resources and is often used interchangeably with the term *usability*. One important accessibility factor is ease of travel to and from the resources as well as the ease of using the resources and equipment. An accessible resource is one that is easy to approach and use; one with little or no traffic en route; one that has adequate, convenient parking; and one that is accessible via inexpensive, convenient, and pleasant public transportation. In contrast, an inaccessible resource may have no readily available public transportation, inconvenient or no parking, equipment that is difficult to understand and use, or long lines for entry and equipment use. Cost is another important accessibility factor that can influence physical activity resource use, particularly among populations of lower socioeconomic status and children and adolescents.

Accessibility is a factor in determining whether people use physical activity resources and ultimately in whether they do physical activity. Research has indicated that children and adolescents with access to physical activity resources and physical activity programs are more physically active than those without access (Allison et al., 2005; Dwyer et al., 2006; Mota, Almeida, Santos, & Ribeiro, 2005). In addition, it's important to note that populations of lower socioeconomic status typically have more limited access to physical activity resources. This is important because reduced access to physical activity resources is associated with increased body fat and BMI in low-income, minority populations (Heinrich et al., 2008). As a result, it's important to consider this additional barrier when working with populations of lower socioeconomic status.

Proximity

Proximity influences whether people use physical activity resources. Proximity can be measured subjectively using self-report questionnaires or objectively using street network or straight line distances. Briefly, network distance is the distance one would travel on streets to get to a resource, while straight line distance is the direct distance between two points; it represents the absolute distance one would travel if there were no buildings or obstacles. The more proximal a resource is to someone, the more accessible it is as well.

There is a strong relationship between proximity of physical activity resources and physical activity. In a study among low-income, midlife women, those who reported greater proximity to physical activity resources also did more physical activity (Jilcott, Evenson, Laraia, & Ammerman, 2007). There is also evidence that suggests there is a direct relationship between proximity to physical activity resources and meeting physical activity guidelines (Sallis, Patterson, Buono, & Nader, 1988). In addition, proximity to physical activity resources may be particularly important for children and adolescents, since most youth are limited to the immediate resources to which they can walk or bicycle.

Within the context of proximity, the density of physical activity resources is another factor to consider. For example, a study found that adolescent girls who lived near more parks did more physical activity than those who lived near fewer parks (Cohen et al., 2006). Similar results were found in women: Women who lived near more physical activity resources and parks were more physically active than those who lived near fewer physical activity resources and parks (Jilcott et al., 2007; Norman et al., 2006; Lee et al., 2007).

The findings from these studies stress the importance of proximity to physical activity resources. Furthermore, these studies suggest that the built environment plays a vital role in resident health and that careful community planning can affect the health of residents. Research has shown that having a nearby park or gym may help to buffer the relationship between lower socioeconomic status and engaging in less physical activity (Lee et al., 2007). As a result, creating a variety of opportunities for recreation and physical activity that are easily accessible can provide a means to increase the amount of energy expended by Americans, a crucial part of solving the obesity epidemic (figure 5.1).

Safety

Safety is freedom from danger, risk, and injury, and it plays a crucial role in determining whether physical activity resources are used. Safety can act as a motivator or a barrier to being physically active. For example, trails and walking paths may offer a feeling of personal safety because they are traditionally placed far away from cars and traffic and because they typically offer more privacy than other types of physical activity resources (Gobster & Dickhut, 1995). On the other hand, safety is most often cited as a deterrent to using physical activity resources (King et al., 2000). For example, crime and traffic are common safety concerns that prevent people from being physically active in outdoor recreation facilities (Molnar, Gortmaker, Bull, & Buka, 2004).

Playgrounds are an important setting in which children can be physically active. However, the safety of playground equipment, which has typically been overlooked in research, plays a pivotal role in determining whether children use physical activity resources. Parks and playgrounds must meet regulatory

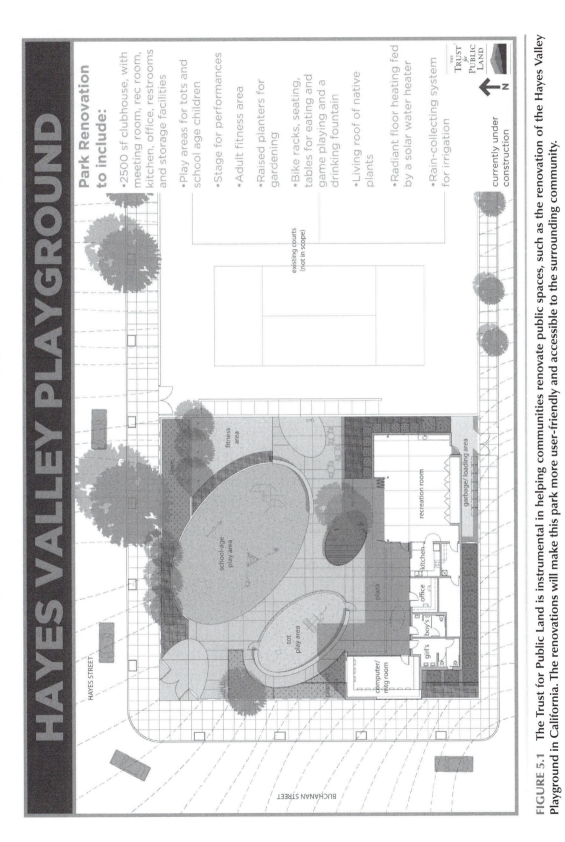

HAYES VALLEY PLAYGROUND

Park Renovation to include:

- 2500 sf clubhouse, with meeting room, rec room, kitchen, office, restrooms and storage facilities
- Play areas for tots and school age children
- Stage for performances
- Adult fitness area
- Raised planters for gardening
- Bike racks, seating, tables for eating and game playing and a drinking fountain
- Living roof of native plants
- Radiant floor heating fed by a solar water heater
- Rain-collecting system for irrigation

existing courts (not in scope)

currently under construction

HAYES STREET

BUCHANAN STREET

school-age play area

fitness area

lawn

tot play area

plaza

computer/ mtg room

girl's

boy's

office

kitchen

recreation room

garbage/ loading area

THE TRUST for PUBLIC LAND

N

FIGURE 5.1 The Trust for Public Land is instrumental in helping communities renovate public spaces, such as the renovation of the Hayes Valley Playground in California. The renovations will make this park more user-friendly and accessible to the surrounding community.

Courtesy of The Trust for Public Land and WRNS Studio.

67

safety guidelines set forth by local, state, and federal agencies before they are deemed safe for use. Unfortunately, these safety guidelines are not always strictly enforced—older parks and playgrounds often do not meet current guidelines. This lack of enforcement has public health implications: Almost 190,000 children required emergency room treatment after being injured on public playground equipment in 2001. As a result, the condition of park and playground equipment is likely an important factor in parents' decisions about whether to let their children play in parks and playgrounds (Bedimo-Rung et al., 2005).

Some population groups are disproportionately burdened with unsafe areas that discourage physical activity. For example, children living in low socioeconomic status neighborhoods dominated by ethnic minorities typically have fewer safe playgrounds, do less physical activity, and have higher rates of overweight and obesity when compared to children in their counterpart neighborhoods (Cradock et al., 2005; Lee, Booth, Reese-Smith, Regan, & Howard, 2005).

Features, Amenities, Aesthetics, and Incivilities

The mere presence of physical activity resources is not the only determinant of their use; the availability and quality of features are important as well. *Features* are specific elements of resources that encourage physical activity. As an example, a baseball field is a feature that encourages users to play baseball or engage in some other types of physical activity. Features can be extremely influential in terms of the types of users they attract and in the amount of maintenance required for the physical activity resource. For example, parks with basketball courts may draw more young users, while parks with swimming pools may draw more families and adult users. However, features such as baseball fields and swimming pools require more maintenance and upkeep than features with fewer, less sophisticated features.

Features that encourage the use of physical activity resources, but are not specifically related to physical activity, are called *amenities*. Amenities add comfort or convenience that may influence people to visit the resource. For example, restrooms, lighting, drinking fountains, and benches are amenities that may be found in a park or along walking trails and that may influence whether people visit the park or trail. Research has shown that people are more likely to use physical activity resources with amenities than those without them (Shores & West, 2008). In addition, research has indicated that the quantity and quality of amenities at physical activity resources may be associated with the prevalence of obesity (Heinrich et al., 2008). As a result, it's important that health-conscious community planners include amenities when building or renovating physical activity resources.

Aesthetics refers to the quality, condition, and appeal of the physical activity resource and its features and can strongly influence whether a physical activity resource is used. For example, park users are more likely to visit a park with pleasant landscaping, appealing amenities, and well-maintained features. Research has shown that well-maintained amenities and features are associated with physical activity (Owen, Humpel, Leslie, Bauman, & Sallis, 2004). As a result, physical activity resources that are poorly maintained, worn down, or in disrepair will dissuade users and contribute to the obesogenic environment.

Incivilities are elements of physical activity resources that reduce the pleasure associated with their use. Examples of incivilities are auditory annoyances, broken glass, dog refuse, graffiti, litter, evidence of alcohol use, and other unpleasantries that could deter the use of a physical activity resource. It should be noted that incivilities are not created as part of the physical activity resource; they are created by users who do not consider the impact on others of the incivilities they create. In addition, incivilities may be considered a source of social disorder

Other than renovating physical activity resources, what strategies can be used to ensure that physical activity resources are used by community residents?

that can contribute to feelings of unhappiness and a lack of safety (Sampson & Raudenbush, 2004); incivilities are also associated with many poor health outcomes (Lee et al., 2005). There is no question that incivilities can deter people from using physical activity resources.

Having physical activity resources nearby, accessible, and available are good first steps toward a neighborhood that promotes physical activity among its residents. However, for most physical activity resources, the determination of whether and how they are used is much more complicated. Factors related to the accessibility of physical activity resources, along with physical activity resource features, amenities, incivilities, and aesthetics are also important to consider.

Measuring Physical Activity Resources

Ever more research is being conducted to examine the relationship among characteristics of the neighborhood built environment and physical activity and obesity. As just discussed, access to physical activity resources is strongly correlated with physical activity. However, access to these resources is not the only factor determining their use. As a result, audit tools are needed to assess various aspects of physical activity resources, such the availability and quality of features and amenities, the presence and quantity of incivilities, and safety and aesthetics.

Several instruments have been created to assess physical activity resources. A detailed discussion of instruments is beyond the scope of this chapter. In particular, we chose not to focus on GIS-based measures because, other than determining where physical activity resources are located—and thus examining factors such as proximity and density—little information can be obtained through the use GIS-based measures. Instead, the following section focuses on three observational assessment instruments.

Measurement Instruments

The Physical Activity Resource Assessment (PARA) is an instrument that trained auditors use when assessing physical activity resources (figure 5.2). The PARA instrument is used to capture information about the type of resource, its size, cost, hours of operation, and its available features, amenities, and incivilities. The PARA documents the presence and quality of 13 features, including basketball courts, soccer fields, play equipment, and tennis courts, and 12 amenities, including bathrooms, benches, drinking fountains, and trash containers. The PARA also documents the presence and quantity of 12 incivilities, including dog refuse, evidence of alcohol use, graffiti or tagging, litter, and vandalism. The PARA is a quick and simple form of assessing physical activity resources that can easily be used by researchers and laypeople alike. The PARA was found to be reliable and valid in evaluating publicly available

1) Date _____	2) Data col _____	3) HD/PA Resource ID _____		
4) Time start:_____ stop:_____	5) Phone Call departure:_____ arrival:_____			
6) Type of Resource 1 fitness club 2 park 3 sport facility 4 trail 5 community center 6 church 7 school 8 combination _____		7) Approximate Size: 1 sm 2 med 3 lg		
		8) Capacity (indoor) _____		
		9) Cost 1 Free 2 Pay at the door 3 Pay for only certain programs 4 Other _____		
10) Hours a) open _____ b) close _____				
11) Signage – Hours yes ☐ no ☐		12) Signage – Rules yes ☐ no ☐		

Feature	Rating				Amenity	Rating			
13) Baseball field	0	1	2	3	26) Access Points	0	1	2	3
14) Basketball courts	0	1	2	3	27) Bathrooms	0	1	2	3
15) Soccer field	0	1	2	3	28) Benches	0	1	2	3
16) Bike Rack	0	1	2	3	29) Drinking fountain	0	1	2	3
17) Exercise Stations	0	1	2	3	30) Fountains	0	1	2	3
18) Play equipment	0	1	2	3	31) Landscaping efforts	0	1	2	3
19) Pool > 3 ft deep	0	1	2	3	32) Lighting	0	1	2	3
20) Sandbox	0	1	2	3	33) Picnic tables shaded	0	1	2	3
21) Sidewalk	0	1	2	3	34) Picnic tables no-shade	0	1	2	3
22) Tennis courts	0	1	2	3	35) Shelters	0	1	2	3
23) Trails – running/biking	0	1	2	3	36) Shower/Locker room	0	1	2	3

FIGURE 5.2 A portion of the PARA instrument.

Used with permission of Rebecca Lee.

physical activity resources in urban and suburban neighborhoods (Lee et al., 2005; McAlexander, Banda, McAlexander, & Lee, 2009).

The Environmental Assessment of Public Recreation Spaces (EAPRS) instrument is used to comprehensively characterize the physical environment within parks and playgrounds (Saelens et al., 2006). The EAPRS is a comprehensive instrument that assesses several features and amenities, including trails and paths, playgrounds, sports fields and courts, special use areas (e.g., open spaces, picnic areas, camping sites), restrooms, trash cans, and bike racks. Although some have criticized the instrument as being too detailed (the audit tool is 59 pages in length) and thus time intensive to administer, it is both reliable and valid.

Last, with the increased popularity of trails for walking, bicycling, and engaging in other forms of physical activity, the Path Environment Audit Tool (PEAT) was created for evaluating trail characteristics (Troped et al., 2006). The PEAT assesses three general content areas of trails, design features, amenities, maintenance, and aesthetics. The proximal neighborhood environment (e.g., commercial destinations) is also assessed.

Variation of Resources by Neighborhood Characteristics

Neighborhood socioeconomic status, density, and other factors may contribute to and explain the distribution and quality of physical activity resources that may, in turn, affect the behaviors and health of residents. Research has shown that when compared to higher socioeconomic status neighborhoods, neighborhoods of lower socioeconomic status have fewer physical activity resources (Estabrooks, Lee, & Gyurcsik, 2003; Powell, Slater, Chaloupka, & Harper, 2006). In addition, neighborhoods of low socioeconomic status have fewer free-for-use physical activity resources than those of high socioeconomic status. These findings suggest that even if they wanted to do physical activity, people living in lower socioeconomic status neighborhoods would find it difficult to do so.

Additional research has found that in lower socioeconomic status neighborhoods where there are physical activity resources present, these may be of poorer quality (Kamphuis et al., 2009). Many lower socioeconomic status neighborhoods tend to have physical activity resources with fewer features and amenities, features and amenities of lower quality, and more incivilities when compared to higher socioeconomic status neighborhoods. These findings, taken together with the earlier discussion of the effect of amenities, incivilities, and aesthetics on physical activity, may point to additional factors beyond proximity that can influence physical activity resource use. Strategies and methods of increasing the use of physical activity resources for physical activity should

What strategies can be used to ensure that physical activity resources, those newly built or renovated, will remain in good condition and will be used?

focus on ongoing and sustainable maintenance and renovation in addition to simply building new resources.

Differences in Rural and Urban Communities

Surveillance data indicate that disparities exist across geographic regions: Rural populations do less physical activity and have a greater prevalence of obesity than their suburban and urban counterparts (Eberhardt & Pamuk, 2004; Martin et al., 2005; CDC, 2007a; CDC, 2007b; Reis et al., 2004). In addition, rural populations are at a greater risk for mortality and experience a greater prevalence of adverse health conditions such as type 2 diabetes, cardiovascular disease (CVD), and some cancers (Eberhardt & Pamuk, 2004; Martin et al., 2005). It is hypothesized that a lack of physical activity resources may be a contributing factor to higher rates of obesity in rural populations (Powell et al., 2006), and in turn, to adverse health conditions as well. Brownson and colleagues found that rural communities lack many of the common public walking resources that are present in urban communities, such as sidewalks and shopping malls (Brownson et al., 2000). In addition, Shores and West found that park size and available amenities varied considerably between urban and rural parks (Shores & West, 2010). To combat these issues, recent community-based health interventions have focused on renovating and creating physical activity resources. However, we should note that a wide gap exists in terms of the amount of research concerning physical activity resources conducted in rural areas versus urban and suburban areas. It is possible that the knowledge gained thus far may not generalize to rural communities, potentially resulting in ineffective efforts.

Emerging Research and Implications for the Future

Research examining physical activity resources and their impact on physical activity and obesity is continually expanding; however, many important questions remain. First, much of the research examining physical activity resources has been conducted in urban and suburban areas, and it's been suggested that these findings may not generalize to rural areas. Rural areas present unique challenges for promoting physical activity, and from a built-environment perspective, rural communities are constructed in ways that are different from urban and suburban areas. In the past, people who lived in rural areas were often more physically active than their urban counterparts; however, current technological innovations have made rural life more sedentary than urban life for most people. It is important that future research focus on these communities and begin to develop intervention and policy efforts for these specific populations.

Second, a considerable amount of the research to date has focused primarily on the availability of physical activity resources and their available features and amenities. While this information has been helpful, it's resulted in an incomplete understanding of how a variety of factors influence resource use. As a result, we recommend combining data from multiple levels, such as individual-level data (e.g., physical activity, perceptions of physical activity resources), park-level data (e.g., the presence and quality of features and amenities), and neighborhood-level data (e.g., street connectivity, crime, and traffic safety), which may provide a more complete picture of physical activity resource use.

In addition, the building or renovation of physical activity resources in communities offers a unique opportunity to conduct natural experiments examining the effectiveness, sustainability, and potential negative effects of making changes to communities. First, examining the effectiveness of these efforts is important for guiding future efforts to create optimal environments for the promotion and maintenance of physical activity. Determining whether changes to physical activity resources can be upheld, in terms of maintenance and cleanliness, is important for ensuring that efforts to promote physical activity are long-lasting rather than temporary solutions. Finally, to date, the examination of efforts to create environments friendly to physical activity has focused on positive effects like increased physical activity, and communities benefit economically from having parks and open spaces. However, it's possible that renovating and building resources such as parks could result in unintended detrimental effects for communities as a by-product of increased property values and taxes. This might lead to gentrification and displacement of less affluent residents. It is important to balance renewal efforts to provide communities with environments that are conducive to physical activity, not to provide them with short-lived relief that may ultimately result in negative effects.

❏ Identify the physical activity resources in your community, both those that are well maintained and those in need of renovation.
❏ Determine which factors strongly influence physical activity resource use in your community.
❏ Determine which features and amenities are favored by members of your community.
❏ Identify strategies to increase and sustain physical activity resource use.
❏ Identify strategies for maintaining physical activity resource renovations.

GETTING STARTED

Summary

Physical activity resources are any public or private setting, facility, equipment, or program that promotes and fosters physical activity in some way. These resources can be free to use and include parks and open spaces, walking trails, and bikeways. Physical activity resources can also be fee based, including places such as gyms, recreation centers, swimming pools, dance studios, golf courses, and sport organizations. Some resources, such as parks and open spaces, may contain features, amenities, and incivilities that can significantly affect their usage. In addition, physical activity resources vary by population and geographic location: Some populations and geographic areas have fewer or poorer resources available. Last, it's important to identify the resources available in communities and the factors that contribute to their use and nonuse in order to better promote physical activity and reduce obesity.

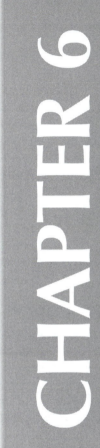

CHAPTER 6

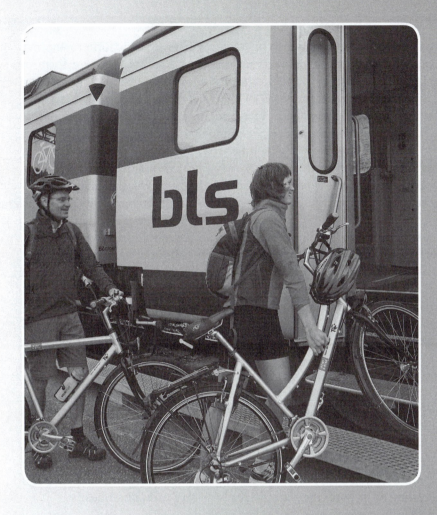

Active Transportation

Active transportation is a means of traveling from one location to another by way of some kind of individual physical activity. It is any form of purposeful, human-powered transportation that has an intended destination (Public Health Agency of Canada, 2002). This is often walking or bicycling, although other active transportation may include jogging, skating, or skateboarding. Often, active transportation may include a synergy of transportation modes; for example, someone might bike from a residence to a transit stop, ride transit for a portion of the journey, and then walk from the destination transit stop to the final destination. A growing body of research suggests that people who live more physically active lives via active transportation tend to have lower rates of obesity (Bassett, Pucher, Buehler, Thompson, & Crouter, 2008; McDonald, 2007; McDonald, 2008; Rosenberg, Sallis, Conway, Cain, & McKenzie, 2006). Despite these promising findings, increasing reliance on the personal automobile is implicated in not only reducing active transportation but also contributing to an environment unfavorable for physical activity.

This chapter describes determinants, correlates, and effects of active transportation. This chapter first looks at the rise of the personal automobile and its association with reduced physical activity. Municipalities that have high rates of personal automobile use typically have lower rates of walkability. Walkability is described in the context of active transportation. Next, this chapter describes public transportation and its role in promoting active transportation, especially active transportation in special populations—for instance, youth walking to school. Last, this chapter discusses stair use and its implications for increasing physical activity and reducing obesity.

Active transportation = traveling from one location to another by means of human-powered transportation.

Personal Automobile and Obesity

The fundamental aim of active transportation is to reduce personal automobile use as the principal form of travel for most people. In the United States, 9 out of every 10 trips outside of the home are done via a personal automobile (Bassett et al., 2008). The advent of the automobile has been a tremendous benefit to humans, because it reduces the time spent traveling and provides a relatively safe and very convenient form of transportation. At the same time, many commuters in industrialized societies have become dependent on the automobile to tend to daily tasks such as commuting to work or school or completing errands or outings. This has become so widespread that in the middle part of the 20th century, city design began to favor suburbs as the preferred residential development style (Ewing, Schmid, Killingsworth, Zlot, & Raudenbush, 2003), resulting in few places to go unless one has an automobile to get to them (Leyden, 2003; Southworth, 1997).

Greater reliance on automobiles is widely believed to be a contributing factor to the obesity epidemic (Cooper, Andersen, Wedderkopp, Page, & Froberg, 2005; Frank, Andresen, & Schmid, 2004). Scholars have documented a similar increase in the amount of driving and obesity prevalence, suggesting that driving may contribute to the obesity epidemic (Bassett et al., 2008). Dependence on automobiles continues to grow in the United States and is also evident in many other industrialized and developing nations alike (Handy, 2002). The average American household has two cars, and nearly all young adults own or have owned a car by the age of 20 (U.S. Census Bureau, 2000). Research suggests that each additional 30 minutes spent in a car per day is associated with a 3% increase in the likelihood of being obese (Frank et al., 2004). The average American spends nearly this amount of time commuting for work every day (U.S. Census Bureau News, 2005). As time spent commuting and distance traveled by car increase, so does obesity prevalence. As a result, of those people who drive the most, more than one in four will be obese (Lopez-Zetina, Lee, & Friis, 2006). About 28% of the automobile trips taken in the United States are under a mile (<1.6 km) in length, a distance that can be walked in 15 to 30 minutes, depending on travel routes, fitness of the walker, and other factors (Bureau of Transportation Statistics, 2002). Holding other factors constant, the addition of one extra walking trip of this length and duration per week would translate roughly to the energy expenditure of 1 pound (.5 kg) of fat lost per year.

In addition to the sedentary time gained while driving, there are many indirect costs of excessive driving. The increased time spent in the car decreases time that might be spent in more physically active pursuits (Frank et al., 2004). It is ironic that driving, originally developed as a time- and cost-saving strategy, allowing people to get from one location to another more rapidly than by walking or biking, has actually led to lack of time and greater expense because it allows us to commute longer and longer distances and times (Tranter, 2010). Furthermore, the increase in pollution and traffic accidents, by virtue of more driving, contributes to a less favorable environment for those who might otherwise choose active transportation (Hinde & Dixon, 2005).

As environmental resources such as fuel continue to grow more and more precious, an additional benefit of active transportation to consider is the savings in fuel (figure 6.1). Increasing fuel costs are associated with reducing driving. However, it is not clear whether this relationship results from drivers becoming more efficient consumers by combining multiple errands into a single trip, or whether alternative transportation options are used rather than personal cars. A related issue is the reality that more fuel is needed to transport more mass. In the United States, one analysis suggests that about one billion gallons of additional fuel burned per year results from an average weight gain of roughly half a pound (.2 kg) per year per person each year from 1960 and 2002 (Jacobson & McLay, 2006). It costs more for an obese person to travel the same distance compared to a non-obese individual. This is not only a personal concern of spending more money at the pump but also a global concern over using depleting natural resources.

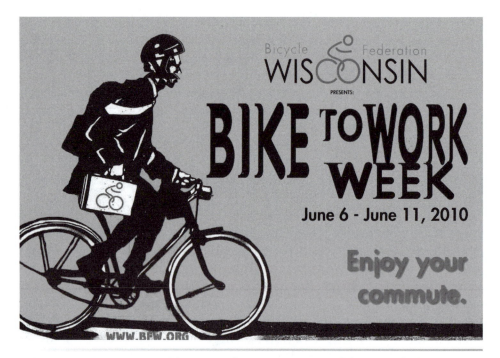

FIGURE 6.1 Many communities across the country sponsor bike to work days, or even weeks as done in Wisconsin, as a way to encourage people to leave their cars at home and incorporate more physical activity into their work day.

Courtesy of the Bicycle Federation of Wisconsin and Firecracker Studios. Bicyclist illustration by Jethro Ford.

Walkability

Active transportation has been related to human-made, environmental factors, referred to as the built environment, that make a neighborhood more walkable or bikeable (Frank, Engelke, & Schmidt, 2003). For example, in Atlanta, residents who lived in the most walkable neighborhoods were 35 percent less likely to be obese than were residents who lived in the least walkable areas (Frank et al., 2004). A more detailed discussion of the built environment is provided in chapter 4.

Walkability is defined by connectivity and density, along with community design that factors in human-scaled attributes such as protected places in the transportation network for pedestrians and cyclists. Residents who report that their neighborhoods have more sidewalks also tend to report more physical activity (Reed, Wilson, Ainsworth, Bowles, & Mixon, 2006). Connectivity is the degree of connection between destinations in a neighborhood (Saelens & Handy, 2008). This is based on the transportation network: A more densely gridded network has higher connectivity than a less densely gridded network. Greater connectivity increases the number of routes between one destination and another in a neighborhood. The more gridded the network, the more likely people are to walk from one destination to another because there are shorter routes, slower automobile traffic, and more variability in aesthetic features that increase visual interest (Transportation Research Board, 2005). Areas that are more gridded tend to have higher density. Density includes the density of goods and services available, but it also refers to the proximity of goods and services. These related factors are key contributors to walkability: People who live in areas that are connected and dense and that have walkable destinations tend to report higher rates of walking (Saelens & Handy, 2008).

Neighborhoods that have high walkability tend to have more physically active residents and lower rates of obesity than neighborhoods with low walkability. People who live in communities that are dense and gridded weigh less and are less likely to be obese compared to people in communities that are more sprawling in nature (Powell, Slater, Chaloupka, & Harper, 2006). The lower rates of obesity in walkable neighborhoods are likely related to the reality that people tend to walk more in these areas. There is a phenomenon in France known as the French paradox, which describes the conundrum associated with dietary habits, including daily consumption of very rich foods and wine, while the French stereotype is one of a very slender people (although rates of obesity have begun to climb in France, just as in all industrialized countries). The French paradox has been attributed to higher rates of daily walking to and from destinations in the beautiful, mixed-use, dense, gridded cities that were designed before widespread use of the automobile.

People who live in highly walkable areas, with many goods and services as well as easy access to public transportation, tend to walk or bike to work more frequently than those who live in low walkable areas with few goods and services and low access to public transportation (Sallis & Glanz, 2006). In fact, residents in highly walkable neighborhoods report about twice as many trips by walking as residents in less walkable neighborhoods (Cerin, Conway, Saelens, Frank, & Sallis, 2009).

Implementing Policy

Wheel 2 Work

In 2007, the northern Canadian city of Whitehorse implemented a social marketing incentive-based plan to encourage residents to bicycle to work during the summer months. The program was developed as part of the official city plan and represented a coordinated effort to reduce greenhouse gas emissions with the unplanned but tremendous additional benefit of increasing physical activity among residents. The city improved existing bicycling infrastructure and created new bikeways for commuters with artisan-designed amenities and safety upgrades. Residents logged the kilometers that they had bicycled and reported them to city officials. To stimulate participation, those residents who reached a set amount of kilometers were eligible for additional prizes. The program was relatively inexpensive and not expressly designed with fitness in mind; nevertheless, it had wide-reaching impact among residents (Transport Canada, 2010).

Public Transportation

A study of commuters in Australia determined that people who rely on public transportation tend to have about 25% lower rates of obesity compared to people who drive to work (Wen & Rissel, 2008). In part, this relationship reflects the walking or biking done to get to the transit stop where one meets the public transportation. People who use public transportation typically walk a total of 19 minutes daily to get to or from a transport stop (Besser & Dannenberg, 2005). People who ride rail, as opposed to bus, tend to walk longer than this. People may prefer rail to bus, perhaps because it is faster and may have higher aesthetic quality and appeal, although it is not known whether people would be willing to walk farther to ride rail rather than bus (Cervero & Kockelman, 1997).

Although many Americans are physically inactive, people who live in denser urban areas, those of a lower socioeconomic status, and ethnic minorities are more likely to walk as a result of riding public transportation (Besser & Dannenberg, 2005). Despite this, those with lower SES and ethnic minorities still tend to report the lowest levels of physical activity (Texas Department of State Health Services, 2007). Urban areas often have better public transportation opportunities, with more transit stops and routes and more frequent trips compared to more suburban areas. High density urban areas are often designed with public transportation in mind, incorporating transit stops and routes into the design to increase walkability and aesthetics and reduce transit operating costs (Frank & Engelke, 2000). The fact that public transportation is easy to use, often less expensive than using a personal automobile, and works best with active transportation to the transit stop contributes to an increase in active transportation in these types of settings.

Public transportation has demonstrated individual benefits of increasing physical activity and reducing individual transportation costs as well as societal benefits of improving air quality, reducing transportation costs to cities, and improving urban design (Frank, 2004). However, many newer cities resist public transportation, and some people believe that it is a waste of money and poses risks to security. Studies suggest that the benefits outweigh the limitations, and many of the limitations cited by those opposed to public transit are not grounded in fact but rather based on stereotypes and misinformation (Frank, 2004).

Active Transport to School

In 1969, over 40% of children walked to school. Forty years later, the percentage has dropped to 13% (McDonald, 2007). This decline represents an increasing decline in daily physical activity for children and may also translate to loss of physical activity for adults, the parents or caretakers who walk with the child to school. Daily walking to school may contribute only a small portion of physical activity in children, but those children who walk to school do significantly more physical activity compared to those who do not walk or bike to school (Cooper et al., 2005). This modest but measurable increase in physical activity may be sufficient to fend off excess weight gain in childhood (Heelan et al., 2005; Rosenberg et al., 2006), particularly when combined with other physical activity opportunities for youth. In addition, children who walk or bicycle to school tend to be significantly more physically fit than those children who do not, indirectly contributing to improved health across the life span (Cooper et al., 2006).

Perhaps the biggest factor in this decline is the increasing distance from the home to the school. This is a product of city development and policies that restrict the location of schools. Often schools are built on land that is inexpensive and not necessarily proximal to residences where children live. Magnet schools often bus children from all parts of a city across many miles for a particular specialized program or curriculum. Children are much more likely to use active transportation if the route to school is less than 800 meters, or about half a mile (Merom, Tudor-Locke, Bauman, & Rissel, 2006; Timperio et al., 2006).

Safety and the perception of safety are also contributing factors in the decision to walk to school (Zhu & Lee, 2009). Safety includes both personal safety, such as the confidence that a child will arrive safely at school without fear of attack or abduction, as well as traffic safety, the confidence that routes will be free from threats posed by automobile traffic. Kerr et al. (2006) found that in a sample of 259 children and adolescents ages 5 through 18, parent perceptions of safety and neighborhood aesthetics were associated with active commuting to school. In a study involving 347 adolescents with an average age of 13, Carver et al. (2005) found that girls who perceived local roads to be safe spent more time walking for transportation on weekdays and exercising on weekends. They also found that parents' perception of heavy traffic was negatively associated with boys' walking for transportation (Carver et al., 2005). Perhaps as a consequence of limitations imposed by safety, children may be more likely to be overweight when parents perceive that there is heavy street traffic in their neighborhood (Timperio, Salmon, Telford, & Crawford, 2005).

Other factors contribute to active commuting to school in youth. For example, residences in areas that are perceived to be more aesthetically pleasing are associated with active commuting to school (Kerr et al., 2006). Parent responsibilities and demands also shape opportunities for active commuting for children. Parental commuting schedules and family structure—which includes whether there is more than one parent or caretaker to shepherd the child to school—also influence active commuting for children (Merom et al., 2006). People who live in lower-income areas tend to have children who walk to school more than children who live in higher-income areas. Although ethnic minority children display higher levels of overweight, they also tend to have higher rates of active commuting to school, suggesting that other influences are involved in their weight status (McDonald, 2008).

The *walking school bus* is a novel strategy for increasing walking to school that has been receiving interest by researchers and community members alike (Kong et al., 2009). To enhance safety, students walk together on designated routes to school along with parent or guardian chaperones. Students are picked up or dropped off at their homes en route. Schools with walking school bus programs tend to have more students who walk to school compared to schools that do not have programs, and those students participating in walking school bus programs tend to get significantly more daily physical activity than those not participating (Heelan, Abbey, Donnelly, Mayo, & Welk, 2009). Participating in walking school bus programs may also reduce excess weight gain in children (Kong et al., 2010), although others have not found this (Moodie, Haby, Galvin, Swinburn, & Carter, 2009).

How can parents increase their children's active transportation?

Stair Use

In addition to active transportation for commuting, travel for shopping, or other activities, there may be smaller daily activities that can be done to increase daily energy expenditure. These smaller increases in energy expenditure may in turn help prevent and control obesity. Increasing walking opportunities and stair use opportunities during the day may contribute to energy expenditure.

Daily stair use can contribute to significant health benefits. For example, daily stair use has been associated with increased energy expenditure, weight loss, fitness, improved lipid profiles in women, and increased bone density (Jessup, Horne, Vishen, & Wheeler, 2003). Stair climbing is easy to do and free of charge, and it does not require special equipment. Taking the stairs rather than taking the elevator or escalator is usually faster and is hardly a perceptible change in a day full of activities.

Despite this barely perceptible change, some of the demonstrated health benefits of stair use are quite remarkable. For example, older Latina and black women who add climbing two or more flights of stairs daily can see measurable improvements in bone mineral density (Pescatello et al., 2002). People who never take the stairs, always relying on escalators or elevators, would notice just under a pound of weight loss annually if they started taking the stairs each time. Stair climbing also is an efficient form of physical activity. Participating in about 10 minutes per day of stair climbing for 8 weeks will result in fitness improvements equivalent to walking 30 minutes a day for 24 weeks. Data suggest that even two minutes of stair climbing twice a day will result in measurable improvements in fitness in as few as seven weeks (Egana & Donne, 2004).

On average, most reasonably fit people can walk up about 70 stairs in a minute. (This is something to try the next time you have to travel to a high floor in an office building—try timing yourself to see how fast you go.) On average this is about 0.15 calories burned per step (Diet Bites, 2009). Walking up stairs is a high-intensity physical activity, with a metabolic equivalent of about an 8 or 9, depending on how quickly one is going (Heaner, 2009). Men expend about 11 calories per minute, and women burn about 9 calories per minute walking up stairs (Calories per Hour, 2009). This may seem illogical since women tend to walk up stairs faster than men do, but men generally have a higher metabolism than women and are therefore able to expend more calories during physical activity and rest. In any case, 30 minutes of walking up stairs burns about 330 calories for men and about 270 calories for women.

On the trip back downstairs, most people burn up about 0.05 calories per step. This is about one-third of the energy expended going up, but after all of that going up, most people are grateful for the easier effort needed on the way back down. Men burn about 4 calories per minute and women burn about 3 calories per minute walking downstairs, and the metabolic equivalent is only about a value of 3, suggesting fairly light intensity (Calories per Hour, 2009). Thirty minutes of walking downstairs burns up about 120 calories for men and 90 calories for women. For both the trips upstairs and downstairs, these calorie counts are averages; individual variation may yield different counts for different walkers.

Two strategies have been used to increase stair use: environmental changes and promotional techniques. In older buildings, built before the widespread inclusion of elevators, people must use the stairs because there is no alternative. Although this is a good strategy for increasing stair use, it limits access to higher floors to those who are ambulatory, and it makes moving heavy objects from one floor to another much more difficult. A better strategy in building design is to make the stairs the focus of most interfloor transportation rather than the elevator or escalator. The flow of foot traffic is directed to the stairs rather than to the elevator or escalator, although alternative forms of transport can be available according to accessibility needs and regulations.

In buildings where stairs are already installed and accessible, several techniques have been used with some success to increase stair use. First, stairwells must be kept clean and in good repair. Foot traffic cannot be directed to stairs that are not safe for use. Second, stairwells must be made attractive. Carpeting or nice flooring may be installed, music can be piped in, climate controls must be implemented, and artwork or other visual stimulation may be included to improve the ambiance of the stairwell. As well, stairwells must be clearly indicated, with signs posted to direct foot traffic to stairs.

Once the stairs are in place, in good working order, and pleasant, promotional messages at the point of decision to take the stairs (versus an elevator or escalator; figure 6.2) may be used to stimulate trial and use of stairs (Eves, Webb, & Mutrie, 2006; Webb & Eves, 2007a). Targeting messages to specific audiences may be useful, as well as using messages from a credible source (Yancey et al., 2004). For example, a health care professional may be a

Why "weight" for the elevator?

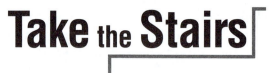

Burn some extra calories.

Take the Stairs

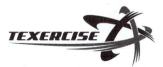

Developed and promoted by the Texas Department of Aging and Disability Services

FIGURE 6.2 Sample stair use point-of-decision sign.

Courtesy of the Texas Department of Aging and Disability Services.

credible source for promoting stair use for people who wish to reduce their risk of obesity and heart disease. Other research has suggested that the message itself may be less important than its placement. Signs, posters, banners, or messages on the stair itself can all be useful, as long as the pedestrian can see the sign (Olander, Eves, & Puig-Ribera, 2008; Webb & Eves, 2005). These kinds of point-of-decision strategies with stair-climbing messages may have transient benefits even after the signs are removed (Webb & Eves, 2007a; 2007b), but it is not clear how long these benefits will last (Nomura, Yoshimoto, Akezaki, & Sato, 2009; Sallis, Bauman, & Pratt, 1998).

> How can worksites increase stair use as a strategy to increase employee physical activity?

Another message for a different audience might be delivered by a peer to demonstrate the time-saving benefits of taking the stairs rather than waiting for the elevator. The message may be delivered through multiple channels to have the maximum reach. E-mail or other electronic communication can be used to promote stair climbing. Previous theorists have suggested that the lack of evidence of sustainability as well as insufficient analyses of the cost-effectiveness of point-of-decision messages hamper broad policy adoption

(Kahn et al., 2002; Soler et al., 2010). Another consideration is that nearly all of the research addressing stair climbing has been conducted in English-speaking countries. Some research indicates that point-of-decision interventions may need modifications to work (Puig-Ribera & Eves, 2010), or may not work similarly well, in cultures with other languages and value sets (Eves, Masters, & McManus, 2008).

❑ Define and describe the difference between, and the implications of, sedentary and active forms of transportation.

❑ Describe the importance of walkability in a neighborhood and its relationship to active commuting.

❑ Discuss factors that contribute to the decision to take the stairs, walk to school, or use public transportation.

GETTING STARTED

Summary

Daily physical activity done for transportation or commuting may be an additional strategy that could decrease obesity. People who drive to work or school are much less likely to achieve recommended levels of physical activity compared to those who use other forms of transportation, which in turn contributes to obesity. Simply owning a car is a powerful indicator of the types of transportation that a person will choose. In many places, it has become so normative to drive a car from one location to another that people who walk, bike, or use public transportation may be viewed as inferior, eccentric, or poor. Strategies that increase the normalcy of active transportation via point-of-decision prompts, walking school buses, and additional incentives or stimuli to use active or public transit are needed. In addition, neighborhoods and environments may need modification to provide a suitable and safe location for active transport. Active transportation is promising as part of a coordinated strategy to reduce the obesity epidemic in both youth and adults alike.

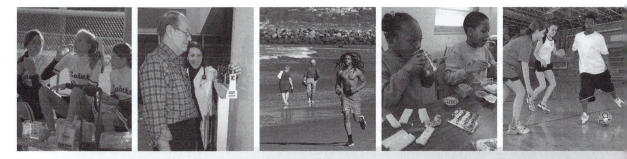

Food Accessibility

The consumption of food, in all its healthy and unhealthy per-mutations, is one of the enduring necessities and joys of human life. However, eating can also be an indulgence, and unlike many other indulgences—tobacco, alcohol, heroin—that can harm our health, humans need food to survive. Food is also important in more symbolic ways, having evolved as important to celebrations of life and hope. Obtaining the food necessary for these facets of our lives has been altered considerably as food technology and supply moved from self-production of food to a market economy. This part of the book discusses food supply, food security, and food technology, offering a perspective on the nutrition transition. In the past, having a reliable food supply was a cause for concern; however, those days are nearly over. There still are places on the globe where finding something to eat is a day-to-day challenge. However, our technological advances, reflected on the menu of any common fast food restaurant, have taken us to the point where theoretically, there is enough food for every person on our planet. The dark side to this tremendous accomplishment is the reality that most of these calories are cheaply produced, making food that is high in calories but low in nutritional quality. It is now, more than ever, easy to consume enough calories for a full day in a single sitting without getting adequate nutrients. The examples in this part of the book have strong ties to policy, and readers will see connections in other parts of this book.

PART

three

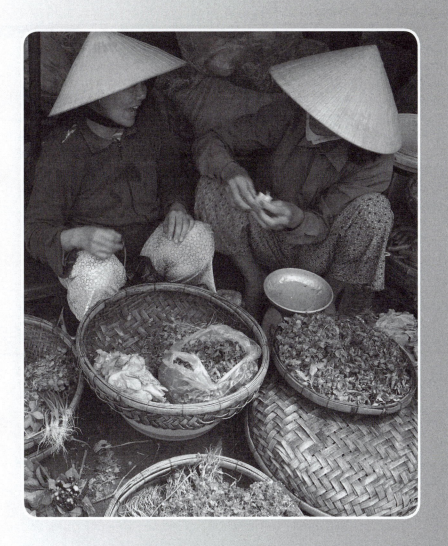

CHAPTER 7

Food Supply and Security

The food supply has changed over the past century, reflecting innovation in technology, trade agreements, and public preferences. As a consequence, dietary habits have changed. Some of this is reflected in the nutrition transition, but it is also seen in generally decreasing numbers of the undernourished and increasing numbers of overweight and obesity. In some cases, these co-occur as a paradox of both undernutrition and obesity. Solutions to this paradox are challenging because the current food supply and consumption patterns have evolved through a complex set of interacting, international policies and preferences. This chapter explores the interplay between the food supply and food security and their relationship to obesity.

Nutrition Transition

Throughout the industrialized world, technological innovation has improved the ability of the food industry to provide access to inexpensive food to more and more people. However, much of this inexpensive food relies on high fat or heavily sweetened products, making a diet that is calorie rich and nutrient poor. This phenomenon reflects changes in the food supply and has been called the nutrition transition (figure 7.1) (Hawkes, 2006). Price increases in energy-dense food have remained low compared to foods that are not energy but nutrient dense. For example, between 1985 and 2000, the cost of soft drinks increased about 20%, and the cost of fat and sweeteners increased about 40%. At the same time, the prices of fish and cereal increased about 80%. In the same period, the price of fruits and vegetables more than doubled, increasing by 120% (Brownell, 2007).

Nutrition transition = the relatively rapid conversion in low- to middle-income countries from undernutrition to overweight or obesity resulting from increased consumption of nutritionally vacant foods.

The global nutrition transition has also been blamed on a shift to the Western diet that contains higher proportions of meat and dairy, with less complex carbohydrate and reduced fruit and vegetable intake (Dixon et al., 2007). The western diet maximizes energy density and minimizes energy cost by emphasizing inexpensive foods with high calorie content. These foods are known as *energy-dense foods.* This kind of diet contains high amounts of refined grains, fat, and added sugar, which are typically able to stay on shelves a long time for increased storage safety. These foods pack a lot of calories into a small amount of food to decrease sensations of hunger. Because of the high fat and sugar contents, these foods tend to taste good, and they are often easy to buy (inexpensive), store (long shelf life), and cook (heat and eat). In contrast, foods that contain fewer calories per unit of food than energy-dense foods tend to have higher nutritional value. These foods are known as nutrient-dense foods, and they are often more expensive, tend to spoil quickly, and may require more intensive preparation efforts (Drewnowski & Darmon, 2005). The western

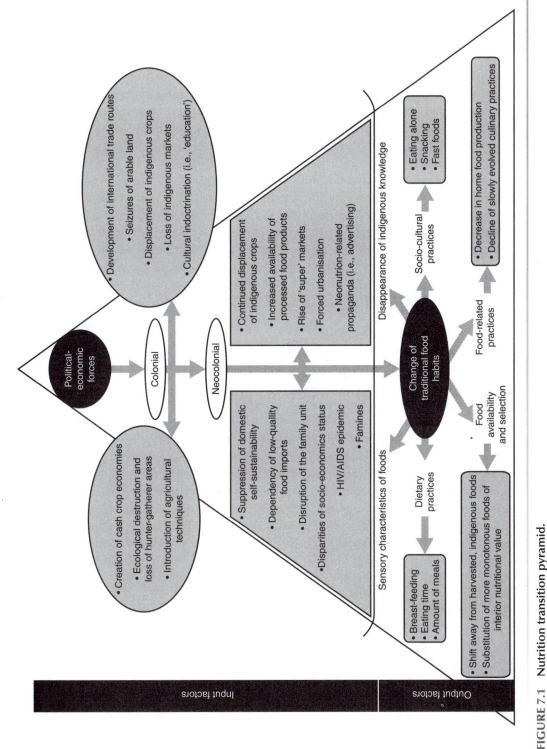

FIGURE 7.1 Nutrition transition pyramid.

From V. Raschke and B. Cheema, 2007, "Colonisation, the New World Order, and the eradication of traditional food habits in East Africa: Historical perspective on the nutrition transition," *Public Health Nutrition* 11(7): 662-674. Copyright ©Verena Raschke and Bobby Cheema. Reprinted with the permission of Cambridge University Press.

diet may provide many more calories than most people need on a daily basis, contributing to the obesity epidemic.

Food Production

The nutrition transition has occurred, in part, as a result of advances in food production. Food production is the creation, growth, assembly, and processing of food and food products and is driven by factors related to environment, agriculture, the economy, and policy. If conditions are good, there is plenty of food produced, leading to lower prices, reductions in compensatory imports, and increases in exports. In addition, excess food can be stored for later use. However, if environmental conditions are not favorable, then food supplies can be affected, in turn affecting the dietary habits of residents. A season of too much or too little rain, unusually high or low temperatures, or even a single severe storm can demolish crops and reduce available healthful fresh foods dramatically. When there are fewer fresh foods available, people may rely on foods that have been stored, often via heavy processing, which can lead to poor dietary habits and weight gain. Poor environmental conditions may reduce crop availability such that a single U.S. dollar might be able to buy 120 calories of fresh fruits and vegetables while it might buy 10 times that number of calories in cookies.

Agriculture also affects the food supply and can contribute to the obesogenic environment (Elinder & Jansson, 2009). Agriculture involves cultivating land for growing crops and raising livestock and is broadly defined to include products both for food and other uses (e.g., cotton). Because many parameters, including environment, economic forecasts, importing and exporting tariffs, and agricultural policies can affect agriculture, there is often a relatively narrow range of locally produced food in any region (Francis et al., 2008; Food System Economic Partnership, 2006). Consumers must often rely on imported and stored food. Imported and stored food is typically processed to endure a longer transport to its final destination. Processed foods often contain additional discretionary calories such as added sugar and saturated fat, which may in turn contribute to dietary habits that may increase the risk of obesity. On the other hand, improvements in freezing technology, in particular, may sustain nutrients for longer periods of time and can help improve dietary habits that may reduce obesity.

Food preferences resulting from individual interests, changing lifestyles, cultural belief systems, or environmental strengths drive much of the available food supply and have created a greater preference for processed and prepared foods. A report from the USDA suggests that most U.S. imports of grain products were processed foods, such as prepared consumer-ready food items and baked goods (Brooks, Regmi, & Jerardo, 2009). Processed and prepared items like pasta, breakfast cereals, mixes, and dough—especially breads and cookies, the most commonly imported processed foods—also typically contain a lot of refined sugar or sweeteners, potentially contributing to poor dietary habits for consumers. Many of these processed foods rely on one of the most common exports in American history—corn. The United States exported $11.2 billion worth of corn in 2007, up 36.2% from 2006 on strong demand from 60 countries around the globe (Woorkman, 2008).

Food production has also changed as a result of the rise of the fast food industry. For example, in the United States, wages for unskilled workers in the service industry have steadily declined since the 1970s. The decrease in wages has increased the number of dual-income families, increasing the number of women in the workforce. Dual-income families have less time at home to cook and eat meals, relying increasingly on prepackaged and prepared foods. The reduced cost of labor, a cheaper food supply, and greater demand for already prepared foods have helped to grow the fast food industry. McDonald's is the United States' largest purchaser of beef and potatoes and the second-largest purchaser of poultry. McDonald's is credited with developing a new breed of chicken to increase production and reduce the costs of McNuggets. Although the food supply contributes to poor dietary habits, a desire for the food contributing to poor dietary habits has also helped to change the food supply. In this example, it is easy to see how coordinated strategies that focus on multiple levels of analysis, changing policies, education, and access are needed to reverse the obesity epidemic (Schlosser, 1998).

Imports and Exports

In the current global economy, imported and exported food is an integral part of a balanced food security protocol. Imports and exports refer to any good or commodity that is traded from one country to another. Imports are products that are brought into a country from another country, while exports are products that are created domestically and sent out to another country that needs them. Most countries import and export food to supplement domestically cultivated supplies. Imports and exports of food are heavily regulated to keep the food supply at home adequate while maximizing the strengths of that country to create profits from excess food that is produced. The balance between the domestic food supply and economic profits is very important. For example, in 1972, huge purchases of grain by the Soviet Union from the United States resulted in shortages in the United States domestic food supply, and unexpected economic consequences resulted from these shortages (U.S. Department of Agiculture Foreign Agricultural Service, 2006).

Food that is more easily traded internationally is often food with a longer shelf life, or processed food, although technological innovations have made it possible for even relatively delicate foods to be traded across large distances. For example, the kiwi fruit from New Zealand is able to travel thousands of miles to be enjoyed by consumers around the world. Although these technological innovations can foster national economic growth, both the quality and freshness of the fresh food (e.g., fruits and vegetables) can suffer.

Much of the importing and exporting of food and products is driven by economic trade agreements. For example, much of the produce imported by the United States is produced by members of the North American Free Trade Agreement (NAFTA) (see figure 7.2). This trade agreement, and others like it, allows neighboring countries to take advantage of each others' strengths. For instance, Mexico has many areas that are warm for a lengthy period of time each year, allowing a longer growing season for some crops. In contrast, many parts of Canada have a long winter, allowing different kinds of plants and animals to thrive. Trade agreements allow each country to share with its neighbors and profit from its strengths while receiving benefits from those same countries in exchange. These kinds of agreements provide greater variety in foods at lower cost to consumers.

In contrast, some countries have a particular strength or specialty that is of interest to countries around the word. Consider our previous kiwi example. New Zealand has practically made an economy on kiwi fruit, in part because the delicious and exotic fruit only grows in very specific environmental conditions. In the United States, food imports for fiscal years 1998-2007 suggest that imported processed foods, spices, and other tropical products have grown from more global sources, with particular reliance on many countries in Asia (Brooks et al., 2009). Sometimes relying on foreign producers is cheaper than trying to cultivate crops domestically. For example, U.S. imports of fruits and nuts have more than doubled since 1998, in part because government subsidies make it less cost-effective for most farmers to grow many of these products.

Although the last ten years have seen a decline in raw sugar products (likely reflecting off-shore processing of raw products), they have seen an increase in candy, syrup, and other products made from raw sugar, resulting in an overall increase in the import of sugar products (U.S. Department of Commerce Industry Report: Food Manufacturing NAICS 311, 2008). Individual preferences for processed food and sugar products continue to affect our national food supply by increasing the availability of these types of foods.

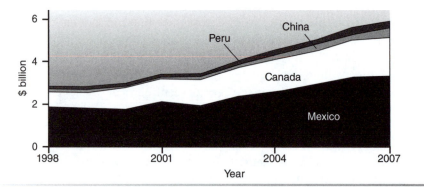

FIGURE 7.2 NAFTA countries dominate fresh vegetable imports to the United States.

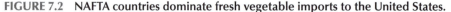

Reprinted from N. Brooks, A. Regmi, and A. Jerardo, 2009, U.S. food import patterns, 1998-2007: A report from the Economic Research Service. [Online]. Available: www.ers.usda.gov/Publications/FAU/2009/08Aug/FAU125/FAU125.pdf [October 4, 2010].

With an increased availability of processed, packaged, and sugary foods, it is more likely that residents' dietary habits and health will suffer (Nestle, 2003; Nestle & Jacobson, 2000).

In addition to product availability, much of the importing and exporting of food is linked to intraindustry trade. Intraindustry trade happens when the cultivation of a crop or product occurs in one country, but some or all of the processing occurs offshore, linking that crop or product to foreign markets (Regmi et al., 2005). The last ten years in the United States have seen a growth in imports of processed foods, which, in part, reflects the processing of products that occurs offshore. Often it is less expensive to export the raw product, have it processed offshore, and import the processed product back, rather than have the entire process occur domestically. As a result of this economic reality, food manufacturing operations are often spread over international boundaries to minimize production and distribution costs. This has the added advantage of being able to ensure a rapid strategy to replenish inventories that may be reduced from food shortages.

The importance of the international collaborative nature of food trade can create problems when there are epidemics among animals or crops that debilitate an entire industry in one country. Concerns about mad cow disease (bovine spongiform encephalopathy) in the United Kingdom, and later the United States, greatly reduced trade for these countries and increased meat trade in other countries separated geographically from the disease. In addition, concerns about the safety of beef allowed the pork industry to flourish because people substituted pork for beef. Sometimes diseases that are not related to eating the food, such as the swine flu (H1N1), can also affect supplies. It is impossible to catch the swine flu from eating pork; however, sales of pork in the United States declined $10 million from 2008 to 2009, partly attributable to these fears (National Pork Board, 2008; National Pork Board, 2009).

Food Storage

Food storage can be a domestic skill as well as an industrial and economic tactic. Individuals, families, nations, and even animals store food. Individuals and families typically store fresh food for a shorter time (a few days) and store processed and packaged foods for a longer time (weeks to months). Countries typically dedicate a portion of food produced to reserves in the form of stored food. This food is kept in case of food shortage emergencies resulting from environmental disasters or economic irregularities that affect the flow of imported or exported food. Food reserves are used to keep the food supply stable even in uncertain times. In more recent history, there has been less emphasis on food reserves as international food trade and production have, to a certain degree, globalized the food supply. Also, if national imports continue to rise as they have in the past 10 years, the need for a large national food supply will correspondingly decrease (Lilliston, 2007).

Nutritional Disparities, Obesity, and Undernutrition

At least partially due to the great developments in the food supply, we now live in a time where more people are overweight and obese than are in a state of undernutrition, a state characterized by not getting enough calories or essential nutrients to sustain good health. This finding challenges traditional efforts focused on feeding the hungry. A study in India found that 34% of the Indian population was overweight and 7% obese, compared to only 6% undernourished (Singh et al., 2007). We have reached a point where we have treated and prevented hunger so efficiently that we now run the risk of promoting overweight and obesity.

> Undernutrition = inadequate consumption of sufficient calories and nutrients, often driven by lack of food supply.

People who have lower incomes and also have less discretionary time available may have little choice but to choose energy-dense foods to satisfy appetites while remaining within a budget. For example, many fast-food restaurants have a low-cost menu with items available for $1 or less, such as the dollar menu offered at McDonald's. The typical item on this low-cost menu may cost two or three times less than other items on the regular menu. Consider a $.99 hamburger compared to a grilled chicken sandwich or a dinner salad. The burger is more energy dense, satisfies hunger longer, and is much cheaper. It is hard to make the case that the chicken sandwich or salad is a better option when priorities are cost and satisfying immediate sensations of hunger. Unfortunately, the true cost of eating these foods is borne out much more slowly, with gradual increases in weight gain and related comorbidities. Recent data suggest that some families living with food insecurity are more likely to have overweight or obese children, possibly reflecting consumption of inexpensive food that is high in calories but lower in nutritional quality (figure 7.3) (Bhargava, Jolliffe, & Howard, 2008).

Another concern with cheaply produced, energy-dense food is portion size. Since oil and sweeteners are inexpensive, it is easy to provide very large, low-cost servings of food containing them. For example, french fries, made from potatoes, oil, and salt (and sometimes a bit of food starch or preservatives), are among the cheapest items on the fast-food menu. It is easy for a restaurant to serve a very large portion of fries and call them a single portion. It is actually the case that the typical medium-size fry serving is about 2 servings of starch (McDonald's Corporation, 2009)

> What factors would need to change in the food supply chain in order to match public health dietary recommendations with the available food supply?

and exceeds the daily allowance of fat and oils (MyPyramid, 2008). Thus, it is easy to overconsume in a single sitting and not even realize it is happening.

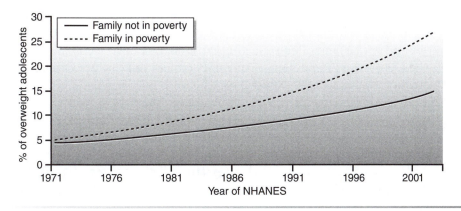

FIGURE 7.3 Percent of overweight adolescents based on poverty level.

In fact, most people will feel happy that they have gotten a bargain for a lot of food and have satisfied their hunger or, perhaps, overeaten. People tend to buy more food when it is inexpensive or perceived as a bargain (Nestle, 2003). Menu labeling efforts and public education may help to reduce the consumption of larger-than-necessary servings of food.

Food Security

Undernutrition is a type of malnutrition that involves a deficiency of one or more essential nutrients. It is generally thought of as a deficiency of calories but also refers to a deficiency of vitamins or minerals. It is related to food security, or the lack of food security, called food *in*security. Food security is access by all people at all times to enough food for an active, healthy life. This includes having access to nutritionally adequate and safe foods and the assured ability to acquire foods in socially acceptable ways (without scavenging, stealing, or using emergency food supplies) (U.S. Department of Agriculture Economic Research Service [USDA ERS], 2008). Food insecurity is typically related to a lack of resources at a population or community level, and in industrialized nations, it is relatively unusual. However, there are times, such as during natural disasters, wartime, and economical hardship, that even the wealthiest nations may suffer from food security concerns. This kind of food insecurity results from food shortages or the inability to transport fresh food supplies to the affected region, due either to lack of fuel or safe routing (International Society for Plant Pathology, 2009).

Food insecurity occurs as part of the ecologic model's macroenvironmental level related to food insufficiency among individuals. Food insufficiency is characterized by an inadequate amount of food intake that is typically temporary in nature (Ribar, 2003). In 2007, 11.1% of households (13 million households) were food insecure, representing no real change from 10.9% (12.6 million households) in 2006 (Nord, Andrews, & Carlson, 2007). For most of the countries in the world, undernutrition has decreased over the last decade, with the notable difference found in a handful of countries, mostly in Central America and Africa, and often reflecting extreme national poverty and conflict (e.g., the Democratic Republic of Congo) (Food and Agriculture Organization of the United Nations, 2009). These countries with nutrition deficits represent a 9% increase in undernourishment, worldwide, since 1990, while there has been a 12% increase in the food supply during this time (Barrett, 2010).

Many people who report food insufficiency tend to have repeated episodes of food insufficiency throughout their lives. Food insufficiency is related to poverty but not directly correlated, suggesting that there may be many factors that impact food insufficiency and an individual's ability to get enough food to eat.

Hunger is the physical sensation of being hungry as a result of recurrent or involuntary lack of food. Over time, this sensation can become quite painful and may have deleterious effects on the physical and mental health of those who suffer from it. Hunger is sometimes related to food security and other times related to personal factors contributing to food insufficiency and then hunger. Prolonged hunger results in malnutrition and can be quite debilitating, particularly in youth and older adults (Life Sciences Research Office, Inc., 2009).

Food security, food sufficiency, and hunger have only been systematically monitored for about the last 20 years. In the United States, a module was developed jointly by the Department of Agriculture and the Department of Health and Human Services for the annual population survey administered by the Census Bureau. The module contains 18 questions that are to be administered annually in a sample of 50,000 U.S. households. Households living in food secure conditions report no or minimal evidence of food insecurity although it is possible that respondents may express concerns about food availability and financial resources. Households may report food-insecure conditions of two types. The first, food insecure without hunger, is defined as adults skipping meals or cutting back on meals to make adjustments for the family diet. For example, parents may skip meals to be sure that children have enough to eat. The second, food insecure with hunger, is defined as a food intake reduction for all members of the household to the extent of hunger (Hamilton et al., 1997).

Government Intervention

Food security, food sufficiency, and hunger have been long recognized by many governments as issues that could be improved with government intervention. In 1996, international governments came together for the World Food Summit at which they committed to reducing by half the number of undernourished people worldwide by 2015 (Food and Agriculture Organization of the United Nations, 2002). In the United States, Healthy People 2010 targeted food insecure households with the goal of reducing the number of food insecure households by half by 2010 (Healthy People 2010, 2009). Initial improvements in this indicator suggested that this goal was on track; in 2006, 89% of households were food secure. However, this had dropped to 85% in 2008 (Nord, Andrews, & Carlson, 2009). This decrease may reflect downturns in the United States and world economies over the past few years.

Most of the U.S. programs enacted to reduce food insecurity tend to focus on children, recognizing that children have specific developmental needs dependent on a nutritious diet and also acknowledging the reality that the children will grow to be adults (Healthy People 2010, 2009). The five basic federally funded child nutrition programs that provide meals, snacks, or individual foods to children are the School Breakfast Program; the National School Lunch Program; the Summer Food Service Program; the Child and Adult Care Food Program; and the Women, Infants and Children program (WIC) (table 7.1). All of these, except WIC, are entitlement programs, meaning that as long as qualifications are met, anyone is entitled to these programs: All eligible schools, sponsors, and children may participate; there are no funding ceilings; and funding grows with need (Food Research and Action Center, 2009).

TABLE 7.1   Summary of U.S. Federally Funded Child Nutrition Programs

Program	Entitlement	Founded	Operated by	Provides
School Breakfast Program (SBP)	Yes	1966	USDA Food and Nutrition Service	Meals with no more than 30% calories from fat or 10% calories from saturated fat At least 25% of U.S. RDA of calories, protein, calcium, iron, and vitamins A and C
National School Lunch Program	Yes	1946	USDA Food and Nutrition Service	Meals with no more than 30% calories from fat or 10% calories from saturated fat At least 33% of U.S. RDA of calories, protein, calcium, iron, and vitamins A and C
Summer Food Service Program	Yes	1968	USDA Food and Nutrition Service	One or two meals and a snack No required nutritional standards
Child and Adult Care Food Program	Yes	1968	USDA Food and Nutrition Service	At a free or reduced price, up to two meals and a snack, or two snacks and a meal per day No required nutritional standards
Women, Infants and Children (WIC)	No	1972	Public health departments at local levels	Specific food vouchers, such as for infant formula and infant jars of baby meals

Thus, the federal budget is set to support these programs, and little political action can change them.

The School Breakfast Program (SBP) grew out of the original Child Nutrition Act in 1966 and provides cash assistance to states to operate nonprofit breakfast programs in schools and residential child care institutions. Both the SBP and the National School Lunch Program allow the individual institutions to determine the food served to meet dietary requirements; it is likely that the cheapest food available will be used. In the United States, more than 10 million children participate in the SBC program daily (U.S. Department of Agriculture Food and Nutrition Service [USDA FNS], 2009c). Children who participate in both breakfast and lunch programs have over half of their daily dietary needs met during the school year, reducing the burden on families (USDA FNS, 2009b).

Competitive food = food and beverages, typically from outside vendors, that are sold in schools that are not part of the school lunch program.

The SBP and National School Lunch Programs have had good success in demonstrating enhanced consumption of important nutrients both during school hours and after-school hours. Furthermore, children participating in

Implementing Policy

Strategies for School Lunches

School lunch time is an important consideration in many countries. There once was a time when children returned home for lunches made at home, but in many industrialized countries, that is no longer the case. Most schools now expect or require the children to remain at school and often offer some kind of organized meal service or meal time. Meal services have been organized with the goal of feeding children reasonably priced and palatable local cuisine, and recently several countries have begun to consider childhood obesity as an important factor in lunch planning. Mexico has been considering a ban on junk food in schools. There is typically no organized meal service at Mexican schools, so vendors sell food to children from carts. With the ban under consideration, greasy meats, fried foods, candy, and sugared sodas and drinks would no longer be allowed for sale on school grounds. Vendors would need to provide foods that emphasized high fruit and vegetable content, low-fat meat and milk, and water, which might be more expensive if these foods were not readily available for vendors. It's also likely that competing vendors just outside the school grounds would continue to carry the banned foods. School lunch programs that have regulated the sale of these types of foods in the United States have shown improved dietary quality but typically only when competing foods are banned. Nevertheless, this may be an important strategy for other countries to consider, particularly when considering the improvement of food security and a reduction in childhood obesity (Stevenson, 2010).

these programs tend to eat less additional sugar in their diets and consume more milk and fewer sugared beverages (USDA FNS, 2001). However, these findings tend to diminish when competitive food products like sodas and fast food are sold at schools (Fox, Dodd, Wilson, & Gleason, 2009). Thus, these federally funded programs may only work to improve nutrition and reduce obesity when they are stand-alone programs and may not achieve these goals when other foods are added to the environment. Competitive food products appear to stigmatize eating the program food and may send a mixed message concerning the importance of eating a nutritionally balanced diet (Fox et al., 2009; USDA FNS, 2001).

The Summer Food Service and the Child and Adult Care Food Program, like the SBP and National School Lunch Programs, are also administered by the U.S. Department of Agriculture's Food and Nutrition Service and operate in a similar fashion. Institutions are paid for meals served, and children and adults may qualify for reduced or free meals and snacks. The Summer Food Service is available during the summer months when school is not in session, and often these programs are combined with activity programming for children during the day (USDA FNS, 2009d). The Child and Adult Care Food Program is for children and adults in day care, and provides free or reduced meals for them (USDA FNS, 2009a).

The WIC program (figure 7.4) is operated at local levels through public health departments. Federal grants are provided to states to provide a prevention-oriented nutrition program that includes supplemental foods, health care referrals, and nutrition education for low-income pregnant, breastfeeding, and non-breastfeeding postpartum women, and infants and children up to age five who are found to be at nutritional risk. Since WIC is not an entitlement program, not all eligible applicants have the opportunity to participate. States will fund applicants until their maximum case load has been reached based on priorities focusing first on pregnant and nursing mothers and infants (USDA FNS, 2009f). Participation in WIC programs during the preschool years has been associated with a reduced risk of childhood overweight as well as a reduced risk of obesity during adulthood. Current research indicates that children participating in WIC are more likely to meet the dietary intake recommendations for nutrients than nonparticipants. WIC participation has also been shown to improve children's eating patterns, significantly reducing the amount of snacking and the intake of added sugar from snacks, reducing overall added sugar intake and increasing the likelihood of meeting the Dietary Reference Intake (DRI) for dietary fiber (USDA ERS, 2007).

Supplemental Nutrition Assistance Program

The Supplemental Nutrition Assistance Program (SNAP) is an entitlement program that aims to alleviate hunger by increasing food consumption and energy intake. Participants receive an electronic benefit transfer (EBT) card

WHAT IS WIC?

WIC is a nutrition program that provides nutrition and health education, healthy food and other services free of charge to Massachusetts families who qualify. WIC stands for Women, Infants and Children.

WHAT DOES WIC OFFER?

WIC's goal is to help keep pregnant and breast-feeding women and kids under age 5 healthy. To do this, WIC provides:

- Personalized nutrition consultations
- Checks to buy free, healthy food
- Tips for eating well to improve health
- Referrals for medical and dental care, health insurance, child care, housing and fuel assistance, and other services that can benefit the whole family

But that's not all! WIC also offers breastfeeding classes, one-on-one breastfeeding support, as well as immunization screening and referrals. WIC also provides parents with opportunities to talk with other parents about nutrition and other health topics that are important to their families.

WHO IS WIC FOR?

WIC is for all kinds of families: married and single parents, working or not working. If you are a father, mother, grandparent, foster parent or other legal guardian of a child under 5, you can apply for WIC for your child.

You can participate in WIC if you:

- Live in Massachusetts
- Have a nutritional need (WIC staff can help you determine this)
- Are a child under 5, or a pregnant or breast-feeding woman, and
- Have a family income less than WIC guidelines

HOUSEHOLD	YEARLY	MONTHLY	WEEKLY
1	$20,036	$1,670	$386
2	26,955	2,247	519
3	33,874	2,823	652
4	40,793	3,400	785
5	47,712	3,976	918
6	54,631	4,553	1,051
7	61,550	5,130	1,184
8	68,469	5,706	1,317

If you are pregnant, you should count yourself as two.

You are automatically income eligible for WIC if you are currently receiving TAFDC, Food Stamps or MassHealth. (MassHealth members with Family Assistance or CommonHealth coverage are not automatically income eligible.) Foster kids under age 5 are also automatically eligible for WIC.

CAN MEN PARTICIPATE IN WIC?

WIC welcomes men! WIC recognizes the important role that fathers, grandparents, stepparents, and other guardians play in caring for kids. Fathers and other caregivers of kids under 5 are encouraged to enroll and bring kids to appointments, attend nutrition and health workshops, and use WIC checks in grocery stores.

HOW DO I APPLY FOR WIC?

Call the WIC Program office in your community to set up an appointment or call 1-800-WIC-1007. Many WIC offices are open in the evenings and on Saturdays so you do not have to miss work. Walk-ins are always welcome.

1-800-WIC-1007

FIGURE 7.4 WIC poster.

Commonwealth of Massachusetts, Executive Office of Health and Human Services that can be used like a debit card to pay for food at participating grocery stores. SNAP has been available in all 50 states since June 2004. Benefits are only for food to be eaten at home and cannot be used for food eaten in the store, for alcohol, tobacco, and nonfood items, or for vitamins and medicine. Eligibility is based on household size, income, and assets. This program was formerly called the Federal Food Stamps program but underwent a name change in 2008 to reflect a broadening of the program to focus on nutrition, prevention, and education. SNAP is based on the Thrifty Food Plan, a market-basket of particular kinds and quantities of foods on which the food stamp allotment is based. In the Thrifty Food Plan, the cost of food prepared and eaten at home is calculated by gender and age for weekly and monthly allotments. The Thrifty Food Plan and the Federal Food Stamps Program were originally developed during the 1930s to meet short term emergency needs, but it has grown into a large program, supporting millions of Americans (U.S. Department of Agriculture Center for Nutrition Policy and Promotion [USDA CNPP], 2009; USDA FNS, 2009e).

The SNAP program has been very successful in increasing expenditures for food among low-income households; as a result it has been blamed for increasing obesity among people of low socioeconomic status. Data from the late 1980s suggested that there might be a relationship between receiving food stamps and being overweight or obese. However, that appeared to simply be a correlation that has not borne out over time. Data actually suggest that the opposite may be true: Food stamp recipients may be less likely to be overweight or obese compared to eligible Americans not participating, to low- to moderate-income households, and to higher-income households (Wilde, McNamara, & Ranney, 2000). Regardless of these seemingly conflicting findings, the true nature of the relationship between participation in SNAP and obesity is not well understood or defined. Future research and studies will be needed in order to fully understand this relationship (Linz, Lee, & Bell, 2005; Ploeq, Mancino, & Lin, 2006).

- ❏ Distinguish among food insecurity, food insufficiency, and hunger.
- ❏ Describe how the nutrition transition has contributed to the paradoxical relationship between obesity and undernutrition.
- ❏ Discuss the role of government policies and programs in reducing and preventing food insecurity and obesity.
- ❏ Describe how imports and exports in the food supply are important for nutritional stability but can also contribute to obesity.

GETTING STARTED

Summary

The food supply is an important determinant of healthful dietary habits that, in turn, contributes to healthy weights. Adequate food security appears to be associated with reduced rates of obesity. Data from federal assistance programs also demonstrate this relationship, suggesting that keeping a nation adequately fed may be an important part of a coordinated effort to simultaneously reduce both food insecurity and obesity. Having consistent access to safe and nutritious food improves nutrient intake through the consumption of nutrient-dense foods—rather than energy-dense foods—and reduces hunger. The food supply relies on policy and industry, food production, food imports and exports, food storage, and food preferences. Environmental conditions, economic trade agreements, and individual food preferences all affect the national food supply, which in turn determines what residents are likely to eat. It is critical to align efforts to improve access to healthful food with agricultural policies and nutritional recommendations in order to achieve public health goals of reducing obesity.

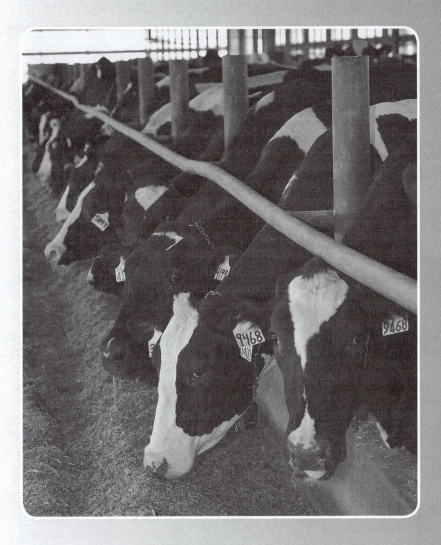

CHAPTER 8

Food Technology

Biotechnology involves the manipulation of living organisms to create or modify products or processes for specific use according to the needs of humanity. Biotechnology has a long history, originating with the initial modification of plants through artificial selection and hybridization to create improved food crops. It has also been used in other arenas such as mining, waste removal, and medicine. Biotechnology contains four major industrial areas: health care, agriculture, nonfood uses of crops and other products (e.g., biodegradable plastics, vegetable oil, biofuels), and environmental uses. In food production, the use of biotechnology ranges from relatively simple fermentation or other naturally occurring processes to factory farming and more complex genetic engineering and cloning procedures. Biotechnology is now extensively used within the food manufacturing process and has altered the way the world produces, purchases, and consumes food. Like many technological innovations, biotechnology can reduce human energy expenditure and increase energy consumption by providing higher yield and lower overall costs. This increased consumption and lower expenditure can initially seem beneficial, but it can ultimately lead to overconsumption and obesity. Furthermore, biotechnology might make foods less nutritious and potentially harmful to our health, simply by altering their natural composition (Food and Agriculture Organization of the United Nations, 2000; Oeschger & Silva, 2007).

> Biotechnology = the result of integrating engineering, technology, and medicine with the biologic sciences.

Genetic Engineering

In genetic engineering, selected genes are transferred from one organism to another. Genes may be from similar or different species. This kind of genetic mixing occurs all the time in nature, such as when humans reproduce. A child has some traits from each parent; the child is a genetic mix drawn from each parent. In genetic engineering, some genetic mixes are simply a replication of what occurs in nature, while other genetic mixes are finely selected to achieve an improved or altered end product (WHO, 2009b).

Genes from any source can be incorporated into any genome. A genome is the entirety of genetic material carried by an organism (Human Genome Project, 2008). Enzyme systems found in bacteria allow the isolation and mass production of genes and the incorporation of these genes into another organism's genome. This system is different from naturally occurring genetic alteration or mutation because it creates an organism in which the DNA has been altered in a way that does not occur naturally. Genetic engineering has been used to develop and grow genetically modified food crops like corn and soybeans. The initial goal of genetic modification of food crops was to increase crop protection against pests and to enhance the ability to tolerate herbicides, in turn improving the reliability and economy of the food supply (Center for Food Safety, 2009).

Crop Biotechnology

Crops that are developed using biotechnology have tremendous insect resistance. Insects can quickly destroy crops, so insect resistance is highly desirable. *Bacillus thuringiensis* is the bacterial source of the gene for toxin production used to incorporate protection against insects. This bacterium is toxic if consumed by insects but is generally and legally regarded as safe for human consumption (Sharma, Sharma, Seetharama, & Ortiz, 2000). There is some controversy concerning the use of bacteria for insect resistance in crops that are being grown for human consumption. The Center for Food Safety seeks stricter regulation, commercialization, testing, and labeling of genetically engineered crops because of potential health risks. In addition to making the crops resistant to the insect, crops with this bacterial toxin gene need less insecticide to ward off pests, leading to lower growing costs (Center for Food Safety, 2009), and lower growing costs make food less expensive for consumers.

Crops have also been genetically modified to resist common plant viruses. Plants can be made resistant to viruses by introducing a gene from certain viruses that cause disease in plants. The plants are then immune or less susceptible to the virus, assuming the virus doesn't mutate. This kind of genetic manipulation is analogous to inoculating the plant against the virus and has been very effective at reducing plant viruses (Johnson, Strom, & Grillo, 2007; United States Department of Agriculture Economic Research Service [USDA ERS], 2009).

It is important for crops to withstand herbicides so that they are not killed by the herbicide that is used to kill weeds or other competing plants inadvertently growing in fields. Weeds compete for the same resources that crops need—water, soil nutrients, and sunlight—and will reduce crop yields and profits if they are left to grow. Human intervention and manipulation of the agricultural environment and the crops themselves ensure that crops will succeed over weeds and nuisance plants.

Genetically Modified Foods

Genetically modified foods have only been available commercially in the United States since the mid-1990s; however, their popularity has grown rapidly. The acreage devoted to genetically modified crops in the United States and elsewhere doubled between the years 1999 and 2005 (figure 8.1) (Fernandez-Cornejo & Caswell, 2006).

The majority of consumers eat genetically modified foods without knowing it. In the United States, most of the genetically modified crops are soybeans, cotton, maize and corn, and potatoes, foods that are now inexpensive to produce and important ingredients in many mass-produced snack, convenience, and fast foods. Many people do not know that they are eating genetically modified foods, because it is so widespread, and there are few labeling laws. The Food, Drug, and Cosmetic Act, passed in 1938, made it a strict rule that the word *imitation* appear on all labels of foods that resemble but are not the

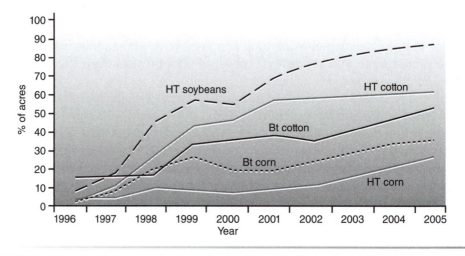

FIGURE 8.1 Growth of genetically engineered crops in the United States. *Data for each crop category include varieties with both HT and Bt (stacked) traits.

Reprinted from J. Fernandez-Cornejo and M. Caswell, 2006, The first decade of genetically engineered crops in the United States (Economic Research Service/USDA Bulletin EIB-11). [Online]. Available: www.ers.usda.gov/publications/eib11/eib11.pdf [October 4, 2010].

same as well-known traditional foods (Pub. L. No. 75-717, 52 Stat. 1040 [codified as amended at 21 U.S.C. §§ 301-392 (1994)], 1938; USDA ERS, 2009). In 1973, this act was tossed out, creating the opportunity for many modified foods to appear on the market unlabeled (USDHHS, 2009). Some scholars have commented that it may be easier to label foods that do not contain genetically modified ingredients, since these ingredients now occur in most foods (Committee on Identifying and Assessing Unintended Effects of Genetically Engineered Foods on Human Health, Board on Life Sciences Food and Nutrition Board, Board on Agriculture and Natural Resources, & Institute of Medicine and National Research Council of the National Academies, 2004; WHO, 2009a).

There has been little interest in labeling genetically modified foods since 1973 because regulations stipulate that food or feed from a genetically modified crop must be shown to be as safe as its nongenetically modified counterpart. It must have similar agronomic (i.e., scientific agriculture) and morphological (i.e., consideration of function) characteristics as its naturally occurring counterpart, which means that it must grow and look the same as it would if it were naturally occurring. In addition, the plant must have similar macro- and micronutrient composition and not demonstrate significant toxicant and antinutrient content compared to the naturally occurring plant (Food and Agriculture Organization of the United Nations, 2004). Most genetically modified foods are evaluated on a case-by-case basis, and if deemed safe, allowed to be used in the marketplace (Food and Agriculture Organization of the United Nations, 2004).

Concerns With Genetically Modified Foods

Despite safety assurances and testing, there may still be problems with unknown food allergies (figure 8.2). For example, a variety of corn called Starlink contains a modified protein that makes it resistant to insects. The Starlink corn was approved for use in animal feed, but not for human consumption, because of concerns about allergic reactions to the genetically modified protein in the corn. Since the genetic modification was not naturally occurring, it was impossible to know whether it would create allergies in humans because it had not previously existed prior to its use in the Starlink corn. As opponents feared, some of the Starlink corn became mixed with corn in the human food supply, and there was great public outcry (Oeschger & Silva, 2007). Starlink corn was pulled from the market in 2000. The U.S. corn supply has been monitored for Starlink proteins since 2001 and has been free of these proteins since 2004.

Another concern about genetic modification of foods is that genetically modifying plants may not only modify factors that improve the plant but may also modify factors that may make the plant harmful. All plants contain small levels of toxins to help them resist predators. These toxins may become elevated when plant genetic structure is modified. In addition to warding off pests, these toxins might be harmful to humans, beneficial insects that do not harm the plant, or local wildlife, like birds, deer, or small animals. As well, these toxins may cause other elements of the food to become less nutritious (Oeschger & Silva, 2007). Factors that reduce the nutritional value of a food are called antinutrients. Antinutrients may contribute to the emerging phenomenon of undernutrition co-occurring with overweight or obesity among those who rely on high calorie but nutritionally limited foods.

There are other concerns about relying heavily on genetically modified foods that do not have to do with human consumption of the plant but rather focus on the ecology in which the plant grows. Perhaps most concerning is the fear of the escape of the modified genes into other species via cross-pollination. Herbicide-resistant crops are a wonderful innovation, but it is relatively simple for them to cross pollinate with weeds, creating offspring weed plants that are also herbicide resistant, muting the benefit of having a herbicide-resistant crop. The same kind of situation can occur in the case of transfer of antibiotic-resistant genes to pathogenic species (Todar, 2008).

It may also happen that genetically modified foods become so resistant to naturally occurring pests that they may overtake the local ecology and become weeds themselves. Opponents of genetically modified foods suggest that genetically modified plants may threaten biodiversity not only by harming local animal populations (as described previously) but also by reducing naturally occurring plants or weeds and overrunning the natural ecology with genetically modified plants and weeds (Food Standards Agency, 2003).

In feeding a population, it is a challenge to balance nutritional needs with obesity concerns while maintaining a viable ecosystem. Expansion and promotion of strategies to increase the supply of and demand for nutritionally dense

Growing evidence of harm from GMOs

GM soy and allergic reactions
- Soy allergies skyrocketed by 50% in the UK, soon after GM soy was introduced.
- A skin prick allergy test shows that some people react to GM soy, but not to wild natural soy.
- Cooked GM soy contains as much as 7-times the amount of a known soy allergen.
- GM soy also contains a new unexpected allergen, not found in wild natural soy.

Bt corn and cotton linked to allergies
The biotech industry claims that Bt-toxin is harmless to humans and mammals because the natural bacteria version has been used as a spray by farmers for years. In reality, hundreds of people exposed to Bt spray had allergic-type symptoms, and mice fed Bt-toxin had powerful immune responses and damaged intestines. Moreover, the Bt in GM crops is designed to be more toxic than the natural spray and is thousands of times more concentrated.

Farm workers throughout India are getting the same allergic reactions from handling Bt cotton as those who reacted to Bt spray. Mice and rats fed Bt corn also showed immune responses.

GMOs fail allergy tests
No tests can guarantee that a GMO will not cause allergies. Although the World Health Organization recommends a screening protocol, the GM soy, corn, and papaya in our food supply fail those tests—because their GM proteins have properties of known allergens.

GMOs may make you allergic to non-GM foods
- GM soy drastically reduces digestive enzymes in mice. If it also impairs your digestion, you may

become sensitive and allergic to a variety of foods.
- Mice fed Bt-toxin started having immune reactions to formerly harmless foods.
- Mice fed experimental GM peas also started reacting to a range of other foods. (The peas had already passed all the allergy tests normally done before a GMO gets on the market. Only this advanced test, which is never used on the GMOs we eat, revealed that the peas could actually be deadly.)

GMOs and liver problems
- Rats fed GM potatoes had smaller, partially atrophied livers.
- The livers of rats fed GM canola were 12-16% heavier.
- GM soy altered mouse liver cells in ways that suggest a toxic insult. The changes reversed after they switched to non-GM soy.

GMOs, reproductive problems, and infant mortality
- More than half the babies of mother rats fed GM soy died within three weeks.
- Male rats and mice fed GM soy had changed testicles, including altered young sperm cells in the mice.
- The DNA of mouse embryos functioned differently when their parents ate GM soy.
- The longer mice were fed GM corn, the less babies they had, and the smaller their babies were.

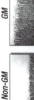

Babies of female rats fed GM soy were considerably smaller, and more than half died within three weeks (compared to 10% of the non-GM soy controls).

Bt crops linked to sterility, disease, and death
- Thousands of sheep, buffalo, and goats in India died after grazing on Bt cotton plants after harvest. Others suffered poor health and reproductive problems.
- Farmers in Europe and Asia say that cows, water buffaloes, chickens, and horses died from eating Bt corn varieties.
- About two dozen US farmers report that Bt corn varieties caused widespread sterility in pigs or cows.
- Filipinos in at least five villages fell sick when a nearby Bt corn variety was pollinating.

Non-GM   GM

The stomach lining of rats fed GM potatoes showed excessive cell growth, a condition that may lead to cancer. Rats also had damaged organs and immune systems.

Functioning GM genes remain inside you
Unlike safety evaluations for drugs, there are no human clinical trials of GM foods. The only published human feeding experiment revealed that the **genetic material inserted into GM soy transfers into bacteria living inside our intestines and continues to function.** This means that long after we stop eating GM foods, we may still have their GM proteins produced continuously inside us.
- If the antibiotic gene inserted into most GM crops were to transfer, it could create super diseases, resistant to antibiotics.
- If the gene that creates Bt-toxin in GM corn were to transfer, it might turn our intestinal bacteria into living pesticide factories.
- Animal studies show that DNA in food can travel into organs throughout the body, even into the fetus.

GM food supplement caused deadly epidemic
In the 1980s, a contaminated brand of a food supplement called L-tryptophan killed about 100 Americans and caused sickness and disability in another 5,000-10,000 people. The source of contaminants was almost certainly the genetic engineering process used in its production. The disease took years to find and was almost overlooked. It was only identified because the symptoms were unique, acute, and fast-acting.

If all three characteristics were not in place, the deadly GM supplement might never have been identified or removed.

If GM foods on the market are causing common diseases or if their effects appear only after long-term exposure, we may not be able to identify the source of the problem for decades, if at all. There is no monitoring of GMO-related illnesses and no long-term animal studies. **Heavily invested biotech corporations are gambling with the health of our nation for their profit.**

Help end the genetic engineering of our food supply
When the tipping point of consumer concern about GMOs was achieved in Europe in 1999, within a single week virtually all major food manufacturers committed to remove GM ingredients. **The Campaign for Healthier Eating in America** is designed to reach a similar tipping point in the US soon.

Our growing network of manufacturers, retailers, healthcare practitioners, organizations, and the media is informing consumers of the health risks of GMOs and helping them select healthier non-GMO alternatives with our Non-GMO Shopping Guides.

Go to **www.ResponsibleTechnology.org to get involved and learn how to avoid GMOs.**

FIGURE 8.2 There is an ongoing debate about the safety of consuming genetically modified foods.

Courtesy of the Institute for Responsible Technology.

fruits and vegetables might be an important component in fighting obesity. It is important to bring policy makers and health professionals together with farmers and growers to determine an acceptable plan that balances these diverse goals in a delicately balanced marketplace.

Benefits of Genetically Modified Foods

There is great variability in the perceived risks associated with genetically modified foods (Peterson et al., 2000). However, when people perceive greater benefits, perceived risks tend to decrease. For example, genetically modified soybeans have been designed to increase oleic acid. Soybean oil that is high in oleic acid is very stable at high temperatures and has been suggested as a means to reduce reliance on trans-fatty acids (described later in this chapter). In consumer surveys, approval ratings of genetically modified soybeans high in oleic acid were higher than the ratings for regular soybeans because of the need for alternative oils. This study concluded that genetically modified foods must supply a unique benefit in order to lower consumer risk perception (Brown & Ping, 2003).

Many believe that genetically modified foods should be more clearly labeled so consumers can make informed choices. Clear labeling would have the advantage of notifying consumers of safety concerns while highlighting health-promoting properties and would allow consumers to decide whether the benefits of consuming genetically modified foods outweigh the risks. However, there is little guidance about how to regulate this effectively (Health Canada, 2005). In 2000, negotiators from 130 countries agreed on a biosafety protocol that requires exporters to identify genetically modified organisms. The protocol also gave importing countries the right to judge whether the imported commodities posed any environmental or health risks (Macllwain, 2000). Labeling is effective only if consumers are knowledgeable about the benefits and liabilities of the ingredients that the label describes.

Consumers in developing countries see greater benefits from genetically modified foods than those in industrialized countries because nutritious foods are readily available in industrialized countries. Many developing countries still have food insecurity, along with malnutrition and economic uncertainty. Genetically modified foods may reduce cost and enhance yield, reducing these problems. Genetic modification is a labor-saving technology that can increase productivity and reduce prices. The downside of this is that, like many technological innovations, genetic modification technology reduces human energy expenditure and increases energy consumption by providing higher yield, improving durability or shelf life, and lowering costs. Although this is initially a good thing, it can rapidly backfire and contribute to obesity (Paez, Zhao, & Hwang, 2009).

The long-term effects of genetically modified foods are unknown; such foods may have improved nutrient composition but at the cost of risk to harmless insects and animals. Genetic modification can result in relatively lower food

Implementing Policy

Urban Community Gardens

Community gardens in urban areas have been increasing in popularity as a source of locally grown fresh food while at the same time teaching community members about food origins (before it gets to the grocer's freezer) and the diversity and seasonality of local fruits and vegetables. Urban Harvest, a small nonprofit organization in Houston, Texas, is funded by private foundations, public grants, memberships, and individual contributions. Urban Harvest has developed infrastructure to help interested community partners start gardens or link up with existing gardens. Gardens are planted in nearly every place imaginable, including schools, youth centers, parks, housing projects, places of worship, and even vacant lots. Urban Harvest provides support for over 100 gardens in Houston and partners with schools and other educational settings to deliver important content on community gardening. Community gardening hopes to increase interest in and consumption of organically grown fruits and vegetables. It also has the added benefit of increasing physical activity, while gardeners are tending to the garden, and simultaneously benefitting the environment. Small community gardens can make a difference to many urban residents by improving the quality of people's diets, improving knowledge and attitudes, and increasing physical activity (Urban Harvest, 2010).

prices for the consumer and economic gains for countries with the capacity to support genetic modification technology. However, the efficiency of this innovation may come at the cost of forcing small farmers out of business and eventually make it impossible to have foods that have not been genetically modified. Coexistence of genetically modified and nonmodified crops may not be possible because contamination may be unavoidable (Curtis, McCluskey, & Wahl, 2004).

Trans-Fatty Acids

Another product of food technology that has grown in its perception of risk is trans-fatty acids. Trans-fatty acids are one of the contributors to the increase in cardiovascular disease in the industrialized world. Trans fat is the common name for a type of unsaturated fat that, because of artificial modification, behaves more like a saturated fat than an unsaturated fat. The modification involves greater saturation with hydrogen atoms, making the fat much more stable; the more stable it is, the longer its shelf life (Semma, 2002). This also results in a higher melting point, making these fats more suitable for baking and frying and allowing them to stay fresh in the pantry in their solid form for up to two years, if unopened.

The process of developing trans fat through the partial hydrogenation (artificially adding hydrogen atoms) of plant oils (generally vegetable oils) began in the early 1900s and was first commercialized by Crisco as an alternative to saturated animal fats and butter. Unlike naturally occurring foods (meat and vegetables), which seldom have more than 5% trans fat, foods containing partially hydrogenated oils contain much larger percentages of artificially produced trans-fatty acids, usually between 15 and 45% (Eckel, Borra, Lichtenstein, & Yin-Piazza, 2007).

Foods Containing Trans Fat

Trans fat is often found in commercially produced baked goods, like cookies, cakes, and crackers, as well as in the shortenings that restaurants commonly use for deep frying. Since partially hydrogenated oil is slower to spoil, it can be reused for a longer time than conventional oil for deep frying, making it especially attractive to fast-food restaurants. Other foods containing large amounts of trans fat are nonbutter spreads, such as margarine; prepackaged foods, like cake and pancake mixes; and fast foods. The longer shelf life makes these foods more economical; thus, suppliers and consumers may be more likely to desire these foods, and that may, in turn, contribute to their consumption and excess adiposity in consumers. Consumption of high levels of hydrogenated oil, such as that found in margarine, may contribute to an increased level of small particles of low-density lipoproteins (LDL) in the blood and increase the risk of heart disease (Mauger et al., 2003).

Limiting the use of trans fat may increase the cost of fried foods and commercially baked goods, which might actually serve as a deterrent to consumption of these types of foods. Although some might perceive this as a Machiavellian strategy, it might have important implications for reducing obesity among those who regularly consume these types of foods.

Often, the amount of trans fat in a given food varies by region since different oil is used in different locations. For example, a 2006 MSNBC story found that McDonald's french fries collected in New York City had twice as much trans fat as french fries collected in Hungary and 28 times as much trans fat as french fries collected in Denmark, where trans fat is restricted (Associated Press, 2006).

As of January 1, 2006, the Food and Drug Administration (USFDA) required food companies to list trans fat content separately on the nutrition facts panel of all packaged foods, in the hope of increasing consumer awareness of trans fat. However, these label requirements do not apply to restaurants, which often fry food in partially hydrogenated oil and serve baked goods containing partially hydrogenated fat. Therefore, when dining out, the consumer bears the responsibility of awareness of products that typically contain trans-fatty acids (Eckel et al., 2007). Health awareness of the risks involved in consuming high amounts of trans fat have led many restaurants in the United States to switch to nonhydrogenated oil for their frying needs.

Risk of Trans Fats to Human Health

To date, there are numerous controlled studies demonstrating risk to human health from the consumption of trans fat. By the mid-1990s, controlled feeding trials and prospective epidemiologic studies showed trans fat to cause an unfavorable change in blood lipid levels, leading to an increased risk of cardiovascular disease. Increased dietary intake of trans-fatty acids and saturated fat creates increased blood serum levels of low-density lipoprotein, commonly known as the bad cholesterol (Clevidence, 2008). Consumption of this fat also decreases serum levels of high-density lipoprotein, or the good cholesterol, which results in an unfavorable LDL-to-HDL, or bad-to-good, ratio (Okie, 2007). The consumption of trans fat has been associated with obesity and an increased risk of cardiovascular disease and death (Eckel et al., 2007). The Nurses' Health Study (NHS) followed a cohort of 120,000 female nurses. Across a 14-year period, researchers found that nurses' coronary heart disease risk doubled for each 2% increase in trans fat calories eaten. The study also found that eating non-trans-fatty acids resulted in a 53% reduced risk of coronary heart disease, as compared to eating trans-fatty acids (Hu et al., 1997).

In addition to changing blood serum lipid levels, consumption of trans fat contributes to the development of heart disease, promoting inflammation and producing endothelial cell (i.e., cells that line the interior surface of blood vessels) dysfunction. This dysfunction is, in turn, associated with the progression of atherosclerosis, the process by which fatty deposits, cholesterol, and other substances build up in the inner artery lining. This buildup is often referred to as plaque and is strongly associated with cardiovascular dysfunction and death. At present, 72,000 heart attacks and nearly 30,000 premature deaths per year are attributed to the consumption of trans fat (Danaei et al., 2009). For the future, it is estimated that if trans-fatty acids are completely replaced in the American diet, between 12% and 22% of myocardial infarctions, or heart attacks, and deaths due to coronary heart disease could be avoided per year (Capewell & O'Flaherty, 2009). Because the risk factors and implications of heart disease and obesity have been linked, a ban on trans fat could significantly affect the existing obesogenic environment.

Feasibility of a Ban on Trans Fat

Compelling evidence indicates that a move toward a diet free of trans fat is needed, but questions remain concerning the feasibility of a ban on trans fat. There are numerous plant oils that do not contain trans fat, such as canola, sunflower, olive, and soybean, and several food oil companies like Crisco have taken steps to reduce and eliminate trans fat. In 2004, Crisco, a leader in oil technology, introduced its reformulated zero trans fat all-vegetable shortening product without increasing the amount of saturated fat. In 2007, they announced that all of their shortening products were reformulated to contain

0 grams of trans fat and have 50% less saturated fat than butter. Soybean oil, which Eckel and colleagues reported as the oil most commonly used in food preparation in the United States, makes up 70% of total edible oil consumption, is relatively abundant and can be found in a low-linoleic form. Low-linoleic fatty acids are more stable than linoleic fatty acids, making them more attractive for commercial frying and baking. Currently, 35.5% of North American edible oil consumption is partially hydrogenated, which is roughly 9 billion pounds. Although this currently does not meet the amount being consumed, it is nearly double the amount produced in 2007 and is steadily increasing. By 2014, it is anticipated that a trans fatty acid-free oil supply will be fully available and able to meet the demand to replace partially hydrogenated oils (Eckel et al., 2007).

Other concerns focus on the increased cost associated with a switch to trans fat-free oils. Despite beliefs to the contrary, trans fat-free oils are cost competitive with their trans fat counterparts. The Holland Inc., a regional chain of 40 quick-service restaurants, reported an additional cost of 6 cents per pound for trans fat-free oil, which they considered to be insignificant. However, others are finding the cost to be slightly greater. Ruby Tuesday, a national casual-dining chain, found similar costs associated with the switch from partially hydrogenated soybean oil to canola oil. However, since its switch in 2003, the chain has encouraged others to collaborate in a concerted effort to demand that trans fat-free products be made available from vendors without an increased cost to consumers.

Implementation of Trans Fat Bans

The demand for trans fat-free foods is increasing nationwide. In 2006, the American Heart Association became the first major organization to specify a daily limit of no more than 1% of total calories coming from trans fat. Since then, Texas schools are recommending trans fat-free foods in their public schools. However, the largest action taken has been by New York City, which passed a ban on trans fat in restaurant food on December 5, 2006. The ban restricts restaurants from using frying and spreading fat containing artificial trans fat above 0.5 grams per serving. Since then, Philadelphia, Albany County in New York, and Puerto Rico have passed similar restaurant bans. U.S. cities in the process of considering restaurant bans include Chicago; Louisville, Kentucky; and Washington, DC. Several states, including Hawaii, Illinois, New York, Texas, and Washington, are considering statewide restaurant bans on trans fat (Manion-Fischer, 2009). Although these cities have been applauded by the health and medical community for their efforts, the American Heart Association is warning other cities who are implementing a similar ban to give restaurants ample time to comply. Without ample time, restaurants could end up reverting to ingredients high in saturated fats, such as palm oil (Reuters Health, 2009).

Factory Farming

Like other aspects of food production and technology, factory farming has evolved to become a major source of our world's food. Factory farming is commonly done throughout the industrialized world and maximizes the highest production of animals for food at the lowest cost. Farm animals are raised in confinement at high stocking density. Animals are considered a part of the factory and are housed in the lowest cost conditions possible. Because animals can be kept indoors, factory farms can produce animals year round without concern for weather conditions. Animals can be maintained in indoor conditions because vitamins A and D, which allow growth in the absence of exercise and sunlight, are already in animal feed. Animals are given antibiotics to combat disease in close quarters. However, every year, we see an increase in the number of salmonella poisoning cases from contaminated eggs, meat, and milk. These strains of salmonella are difficult to treat because they are antibiotic resistant. Antibiotics are not the only chemicals administered to factory farm animals; many animals are fed growth-promoting hormones and appetite stimulants, and their feed is contaminated with pesticides, fertilizers, herbicides, and aflatoxins that collect in the animals' tissues and milk (Ross, 2010).

What would be the expected impact of eliminating factory farming on the food supply and obesity rates in the United States?

Many animal rights advocates have petitioned against factory farming because animals are often housed in suboptimal living conditions and given antibiotics, hormones, and other chemicals to encourage high productivity. In some cases, animals are surgically or genetically modified to reduce the need for free-range living conditions and to enhance tolerance for crowded housing. For example, factory-farmed broiler chickens are selectively bred and genetically altered to produce bigger thighs and breasts. These birds are typically unable to stand, so the birds are subject to the chicken equivalent of bed sores, increasing risk for infection. To reduce the time to market and thus avoid infection, chickens are fed growth hormones and antibiotics, creating a food product that may or may not be ideal for human consumption. Nevertheless, factory farming has increased the availability of low-cost meat, contributing additional calories to the dietary habits of residents of industrialized nations.

The living conditions of factory-farmed animals are less than ideal and may produce animals that are not ideal for consumption, in part because of residual hormones or antibiotics given to the animal. Even with antibiotics, factory farming has long been a contributing factor to human infectious disease (Wolfe, Dunavan, & Diamond, 2007). As well, animals living in stressful conditions may have excess stress hormones, and additional growth hormones are often given to factory-farmed animals to speed up growth. These residual chemicals found in the animal may predispose humans to faster growth and weight gain. Consuming meat, milk, cheese, and dairy products hastens the sexual development of children and promotes weight gain and early menarche (Gunther, Karaolis-Danckert, Kroke, Remer, & Buyken, 2010; Kagawa, 1978; Remer et al., 2010; Saenz de Rodriguez, Bongiovanni, & Conde de Borrego, 1985). Thus, opponents suggest, factory farming contributes to obesity, and health care professionals should recommend greater reliance on plant-based foods to avoid exposure to factory-farmed products (Akhtar, Greger, Ferdowsian, & Frank, 2009).

Factory farming has the potential to increase access to animal protein at low cost to consumers. However, it comes with the cost of added hormones, antibiotics, and other chemicals that may, in turn, increase weight gain and overdevelopment in children. The effects of this are not well defined or documented; however, it is quite likely that the low price tag of factory-farmed animals may come with a high health cost contributing to the obesogenic environment.

❑ Define and describe the role of biotechnology as a favorable and unfavorable force affecting the food supply.

❑ Understand the advantages and disadvantages of genetic engineering and modification of food and its effects on obesity.

❑ Discuss the contribution of technological innovation in food to the health of citizens and the obesity epidemic.

❑ Understand the benefits and limitations of trans-fatty acids instead of saturated animal fat.

GETTING STARTED

Summary

Consumers often know little about food technology and its benefits or limitations because much of the research and innovation has been implemented with little consumer input or government regulation. The biotechnological transformation of America's food supply (e.g., genetic engineering, factory farming, trans fat production) is a scientific and business venture that has developed and profited tremendously in recent years. Improvements in technology can lead to improved food security and nutritional value, as well as reduced cost to producers and consumers. However, many of the long-term consequences of food technology advances are not well researched or understood. Although there are great benefits to biologic and technological innovation, there may be great costs to human health by way of decreasing energy expenditure, burdening the environment, and increasing the supply of food that has high energy density with food that has low energy cost and low nutritional value.

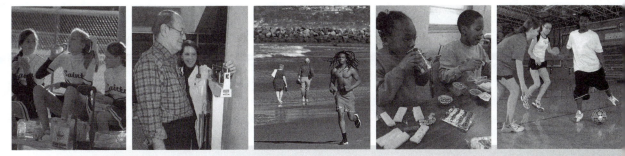

Public Policy, Sociocultural Influences, and Obesity

Contextual factors, such as policies and sociocultural influences, are widely endorsed as some of the most promising avenues for intervention in the goal of reversing the obesogenic environment. The U.S. National Physical Activity Plan (2010) endorses working with policy makers to promote environments that foster daily physical activity. There are numerous policies that influence physical activity and dietary habits and, in turn, obesity. We discuss policies that directly impact individual habits and choices as well as policies that impact environments or other factors that essentially make the obesogenic choice the only choice available. Policies operate within the broader social context that includes cultural and societal influences, and readers will see overlap among these chapters. Furthermore, the policy and sociocultural chapters are interrelated with every chapter in this book in some way or another. Because of this relationship, the challenges of changing policies and working within sociocultural contexts are complex and difficult but extremely important for sustainable change.

PART

four

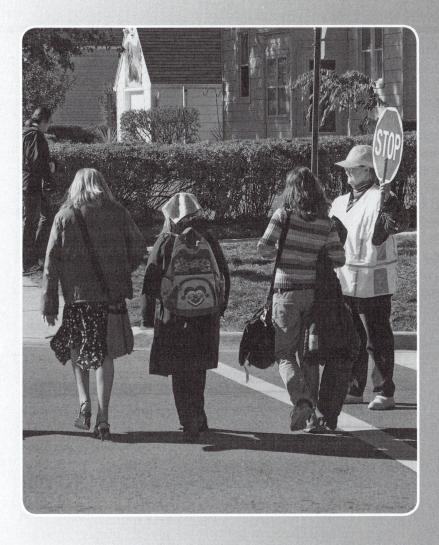

CHAPTER 9

Policy and Individual Health Choices

In 1974, an editorial in a leading medical journal called obesity the most important nutritional disease in the affluent countries of the world ("Editorial: Infant and adult obesity," 1974). After almost four decades, the problem of obesity not only plagues affluent countries but has found its way into nearly all countries and has eclipsed undernutrition as a medical problem (Flegal, 2005; Flegal, Carroll, Ogden, & Johnson, 2002; Kuczmarski, Flegal, Campbell, & Johnson, 1994; Misra & Khurana, 2008; Okosun et al., 2004; Popkin, 1994; Seidell, 1995; Silventoinen et al., 2004). Despite this, there are few effective and sustainable individual-based approaches. Careful attention to diet and exercise has been shown to be very effective in the short term, but it is not sustainable for most people. Broader-scale, coordinated efforts at regulating environments, resource availability, and opportunities, such as policy approaches, have been suggested by leading experts as the only answer to controlling the obesity epidemic. Policies can work at the macro- or microenvironmental levels in the context of the ecologic milieu. For example, government policies regulate elements in the macroenvironment, but this regulation affects individuals by changing individual behavior to comply with the macropolicy. Microenvironments can also have policies—for example, worksite or school policies happen in the microenvironment.

In the early 20th century, in most of the industrialized world, policies concerning safe drinking water began to require that small amounts of purification chemicals, such as chlorine, be added to water supplies, in addition to standard filtration methods. Although in large amounts chlorine can be harmful to humans, in small amounts, chlorine kills microbial organisms and is harmless to humans, providing important protection against water-borne illnesses. This simple policy has saved countless lives over the last century and has improved the quality of life for many. Although some individuals believe that the government should not regulate the water supply, most believe that the good of the many outweighs the preferences of the few. Policy approaches work on the premise that a law that regulates the behavior of humans or the infrastructure in which we live may unfavorably alter the behavior of a few or provide fewer choices; however, in the big picture, the lives saved, health preserved, and greater good achieved outweighs the actions or preferences of a few individuals.

Policy can play an important role in public health approaches to prevent obesity and promote health. The intersection of policy and public health has been a viable modality of reducing the impact of public health problems for many years. For example, policies that regulate immunizations were instrumental in the prevention and eradication of debilitating diseases such as smallpox (McKenzie, Pinger, & Kotecki, 2005). Other recent policy successes have focused on regulating the tobacco industry. Although tobacco products are still widely available for purchase, regulations have been effective in decreasing individual and environmental access to tobacco products for children and reducing opportunities for smoking for adults. Obesity prevention and treatment policies are macroenvironmental factors that intersect with individual behavior by changing the knowledge, attitudes, or behaviors of many. This intersection then changes the behavior of the individual by improving dietary habits or increasing physical activity, and regardless of whether the individual is aware of this behavior change, the net outcome is the same.

Levels of Prevention

In the case of disease prevention and treatment via policy approaches, it is helpful to consider the levels of prevention. Primary prevention is the level at which a disease is prevented from occurring in the first place. In a perfect world, most healthy people would be able to avoid developing overweight or obesity by maintaining energy balance throughout the life span. Since this is not the case for most people in the industrialized world, many approaches emphasizing secondary prevention have been implemented. Secondary prevention occurs after the disease has occurred but before any serious health consequences have occurred. Thus, once someone is diagnosed as overweight, secondary prevention strategies (i.e., weight loss) should be implemented before the situation escalates to obesity or any other health-compromising conditions. It is often the case that the opportunity for secondary prevention is missed, and tertiary prevention must be employed. Tertiary prevention occurs after serious health consequences have taken place, and a disease state is present. At this time, the person has the signs and symptoms of disease, and the focus is on preventing pain and damage from the disease, slowing disease progression, preventing complications from the disease, and whenever possible, reversing the disease itself as well as damage from the disease.

> Primary prevention = preventing the occurrence of a disease, accident or ailment.
>
> Secondary prevention = detecting and treating early signs of disease or injury to prevent disability and comorbid problems.
>
> Tertiary prevention = preventing complications or further damage from established, chronic disease or health-compromising conditions.

Policies can affect obesity at all levels of prevention. For example, policies that help people to eat healthfully and stay physically active can work at all levels but are mostly used as primary prevention. In contrast, policies that help people gain access to healthcare may focus on tertiary prevention. There are also policies developed and maintained for reasons that have nothing to do with obesity but that have unexpected consequences like hindering or promoting obesity. For example, policies aimed at improving public transportation as a means of preserving clean air may also affect obesity by promoting physical activity. Policies that regulate import and export of grains and other crops may affect obesity by changing the price and availability of the food supply.

Many strategies to reduce obesity have focused on individual determinants and individual responsibility for obesity. Individually oriented strategies have grown out of the belief that individuals who are obese do not have the knowledge, skills, or willpower to manage their eating habits or exercise regularly. The challenge of these approaches is that they place responsibility for the obesity epidemic solely on the individual. In reality, the problem of obesity has not reached epidemic proportions simply because of lack of individual effort; rather, the obesity epidemic represents a failure at all levels of human existence and understanding. Ecologic models describe these levels. It is easy to see that pervasive environmental and social influences may drive individual behavior even when people understand the relationship between excess energy intake and insufficient energy expenditure. Some government agencies and social organizations have taken steps to regulate obesity via policy by creating national guidelines, educating individuals, and regulating food purchases. These other policy approaches are discussed below.

Guidelines

Initial efforts to regulate obesity and health behaviors to prevent and treat obesity via policy have encouraged increasing public awareness of the role of dietary habits and physical activity in the development and maintenance of obesity. Policy makers regulate the fiscal support of the government agencies that maintain nutrition, physical activity, and other health guidelines, and this, in turn, determines when and how guidelines will be revised and promoted. Guidelines may be revised frequently or infrequently, depending on governmental priorities. Priorities are not only fiscal in nature but may also be driven by scientific discovery, technological innovation, and industry standards and preferences. The guidelines, in turn, affect information distributed in public channels through policy statements, educational curricula, and industry promotion.

In the United States, government agencies, like the Department of Health and Human Services, the Food and Drug Administration, and the United States Department of Agriculture, offer guidelines both in print and Internet form. Guidelines are developed based on existing data but sometimes are also influenced by political pressures. For example, research over the past two decades has shown that trans-fatty acids that are often found in commercially deep-fried food or baked goods are detrimental to cardiovascular health in humans. Despite this research, guidelines about consuming trans-fatty acids and regulations about food labels identifying them have only been widely available since 2006. The time gap behind the science demonstrating health risk and the enactment of policy that provides information about the presence of a harmful food has been driven by lack of awareness and understanding from consumers and lack of competitively priced, viable fat alternatives in industry. As consumers have become more aware of the risks of trans-fatty acids, and technological innovation has provided alternatives for industry, policy makers have been able to improve regulations to protect consumers from trans-fatty acids while allowing consumers to continue to eat their favor-

Implementing Policy

Traffic Light

In the United Kingdom, a food labeling program called Traffic Light has been introduced by the National Food Standards Agency. It uses the colors red, amber, or green on a label to indicate at a glance how a particular food fares in nutritional content. Consumers are able to understand the amount of fat, saturated fat, sugar, and salt contained in a food (red for high, amber for not high but not low, and green for low). Consumers are instructed to go for green or amber for daily use and red only as a special treats. This system promotes a high level of understanding, regardless of consumer knowledge of particular nutritional guidelines or how to achieve them. As the Traffic Light's labels are not mandatory, companies that have adopted the labels may be more likely to be foods that have greens or ambers; however, even this stands to benefit consumers who are concerned about improving their dietary habits. The U.K. National Food Standards Agency is actively seeking more food companies to promote the program, particularly fast-food and convenience food manufacturers (U.K. National Food Standards Agency, 2010).

ite foods. Technological innovations and consumer awareness are only a few examples of the many ways guidelines can affect individual health behaviors that can, in turn, affect weight status. Educating individuals is a common individually focused policy approach.

The United States, along with most countries, offers guidelines for nutrition (USFDA, 2009a). The USDA Center for Nutrition Policy and Promotion Dietary Guidelines offers dietary guidelines that are issued and updated roughly every five years. The Departments of Agriculture (USDA) and Health and Human Services (HHS) jointly provide information to revise the dietary guidelines based on new dietary discoveries and the changing face of the U.S. population. The Dietary Guidelines for Americans were considerably revised in 2010 (USDHHS and USDA, 2010). The new guidelines have a much heavier emphasis on the reality that many Americans, despite struggling with overweight and obesity, still face nutritional deficits. In addition, the 2010 Dietary Guidelines emphasize more practical considerations on how to integrate dietary guidelines and recognize the role that environmental and societal factors play in obesity. The USDA Food Pyramid offers interactive Web-based consumer education tools illustrating dietary guidelines geared for youth and adults in the general population, with special attention to preschoolers and expectant mothers. Recent revision of the pyramid has endeavored to make guidelines clearer, easier to understand, and more helpful for guiding consumers in planning menus in line with the guidelines. It also includes some physical activity guidelines along with dietary habits guidelines, reflecting closer ties between the elements of energy balance (USDA, 2009).

Educating Individuals

Although simply changing knowledge is seldom sufficient to change behavior, many practitioners believe that understanding recommendations and their rationale is important for individual behavior change. Many school policies have been enacted, with the bulk of the policies focused on information taught to students or on food and physical activity offerings available during the school day. More than 95% of American children ages 5 to 17 are enrolled in school, and information distributed in schools has the potential to affect nearly all children who attend school regularly (Story, Kaphingst, & French, 2006). More information on policies that change the school environment is provided in chapter 10. This section focuses on educational efforts aimed at individuals.

One example of a school policy approach that is aimed at individuals is the Child and Nutrition and WIC Reauthorization Act. The Child Nutrition and WIC Reauthorization Act was signed into law in 2004 to build on the original Child Nutrition Act from 1966 that provided healthful food during the school day. The 2004 Child Nutrition Act aimed to improve nutrition and physical education and to update food standards in American schools. Experts in nutrition education note that 15 hours are needed to bring about change in knowledge, and 50 hours are required for changes in attitudes and behaviors (Connell, Turner, & Mason, 1985). In contrast, the typical school health curriculum includes an average of only five hours per school year devoted to nutrition education, suggesting that merely having the policy in place may not yield the effects hoped for by policy proponents (Action for Healthy Kids, 2009). Future regulation development may be needed to require specific instruction in health behavior and weight management as part of the school curriculum. The 2004 Child Nutrition Act also requires local wellness policies to be developed and implemented by parents, teachers, administrators, school food services, school boards, and the public to improve coordination between schools and other individuals and organizations who may provide care and service for children. Changing the school curriculum is well intentioned but difficult to accomplish. It involves improving teacher knowledge in order to deliver the information and obtaining administrative support for allowing time away from other subjects taught during the school day. These changes, although difficult to accomplish, are needed to improve children's health knowledge for both the current and future prevention and treatment of obesity.

Although it was once a requirement, many schools no longer offer daily physical education in the curriculum because no policies require it. Daily physical education is believed to teach important knowledge and skills for a lifetime of physical activity. However, studies have shown that physical education may not always achieve this goal if it is not taught by a properly trained instructor, providing a variety of options at all skill levels. Some evidence has suggested that physical education can lead to decreases in physical activity if children are placed in scenarios that are too competitive or challenging (Drewe, 1998; Musch & Grondin, 2001). National standards mandate a variety of activities (National Association for Sports and Physical Education, 2004).

Experts have recommended that children receive between 150 to 225 minutes per week of physical education emphasizing progressive challenges and fun. They urge minimizing penalties for less gifted children and never using physical activity as a punishment (e.g., running laps for being late to class). Teachers must be specifically trained in the teaching of physical education, rather than relying on teachers trained in other academic topics. For example, both the National Association for Sports and Physical Education and the National Association of State Boards of Education oversee physical education instructor training and have national standards for physical educators. Policies are needed to increase physical activity during the school day and inspire lifelong physical activity as a means for preventing and reducing obesity.

> What are some examples of policies that have improved public health knowledge, attitudes, and habits?

Regulations at the Point of Purchase

Most consumers make their food purchase and consumption decisions at the retail point of purchase. Whether at a store, a restaurant, or some other venue like a vending machine, most people decide at that point what they will buy and consume based on product specifications, price, placement, and promotions (described in more detail in chapter 13). Policy approaches may be used to regulate all four elements involved in the purchase and consumption decision.

The food industry must adhere to regulations that protect consumers from eating poor quality or unsafe foods. The food industry is required to inform the public concerning the ingredients in food by way of food labeling. Food labeling is regulated by the Federal Drug Administration in the United States, and other countries often have similar agencies and labeling requirements. In the United States, food labels are required for nearly all foods that are packaged or prepared—such as canned and frozen foods, breakfast cereals, baked goods, beverages, and snacks—but they are optional for many raw foods, like fresh fruits, vegetables, and fish (USFDA, 2009b). Some studies have suggested that labels are too complex, making understanding the nutritional value of food particularly challenging for older adults and those with less education, and as a result, labeling has been simplified (Levy & Fein, 1998). Many proponents of more detailed food labeling suggest that if consumers know more about what they are eating, they may be more likely to make more healthful choices. Some evidence suggests that consumers believe that reading labels is an important health improvement strategy, but a lack of understanding about nutrients and serving sizes as well as inconsistency in the labels themselves hamper effective reading of labels (see figure 9.1) (Bassett et al., 2008; Borra, 2006; Burton, Creyer, Kees, & Huggins, 2006; Fitzgerald, Damio, Segura-Perez, & Perez-Escamilla, 2008; Lando & Labiner-Wolfe, 2007; Vari-yam, 2008). Furthermore, even when consumers do understand food labels, healthful choices based on the labels may be countered by the consumption of other less healthful choices, netting no real change in dietary habits (Teisl

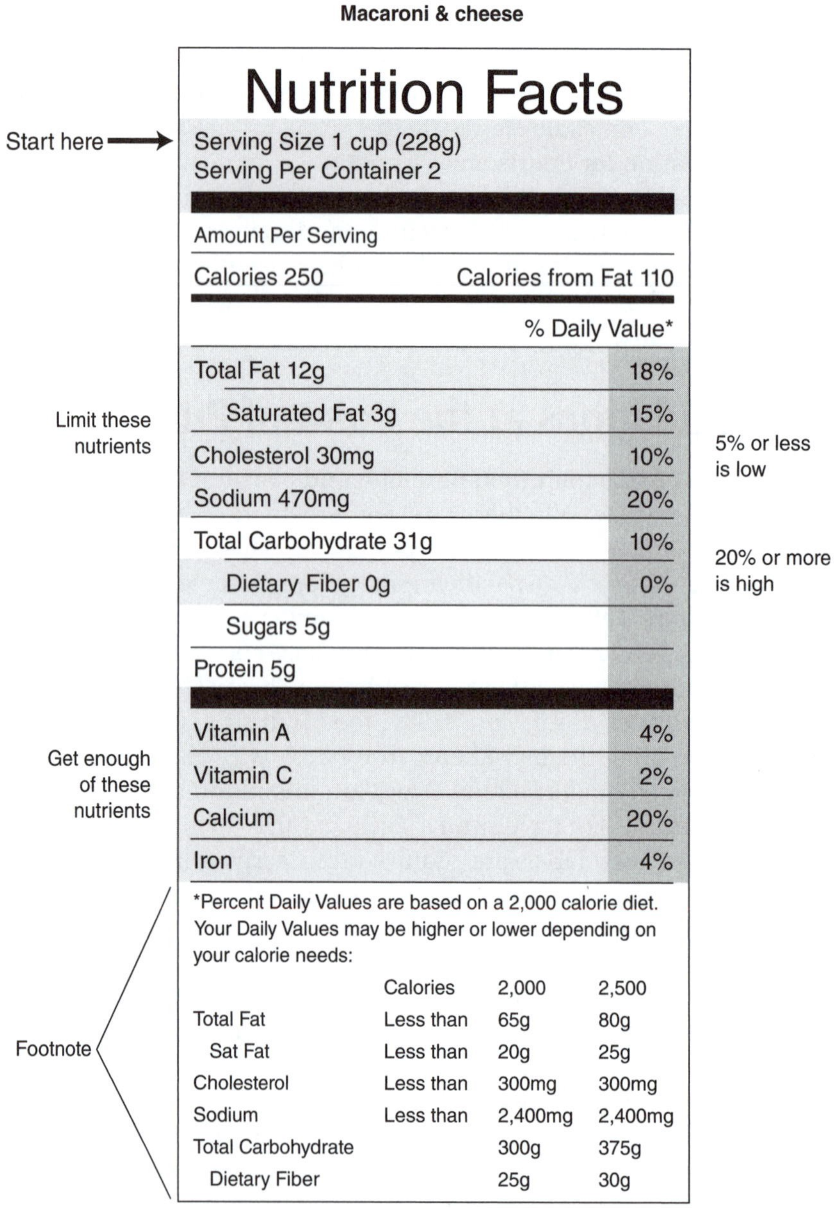

Macaroni & cheese

Nutrition Facts

Start here ➡️ Serving Size 1 cup (228g)
Serving Per Container 2

Amount Per Serving

Calories 250	Calories from Fat 110

	% Daily Value*
Total Fat 12g	18%
Saturated Fat 3g	15%
Cholesterol 30mg	10%
Sodium 470mg	20%
Total Carbohydrate 31g	10%
Dietary Fiber 0g	0%
Sugars 5g	
Protein 5g	

Vitamin A	4%
Vitamin C	2%
Calcium	20%
Iron	4%

Limit these nutrients

5% or less is low

20% or more is high

Get enough of these nutrients

*Percent Daily Values are based on a 2,000 calorie diet.
Your Daily Values may be higher or lower depending on
your calorie needs:

	Calories	2,000	2,500
Total Fat	Less than	65g	80g
Sat Fat	Less than	20g	25g
Cholesterol	Less than	300mg	300mg
Sodium	Less than	2,400mg	2,400mg
Total Carbohydrate		300g	375g
Dietary Fiber		25g	30g

Footnote

FIGURE 9.1 How to read a food label.

& Levy, 1997). Although having a clear and consistent food labeling policy is an important part of making healthful dietary choices, it is clear that this policy must be coupled with appropriate consumer education to be effective.

Recently, there has been a move to require chain restaurants to provide information about calorie content on menus or menu boards and nutrition labeling on wrappers to inform the public about the contents of food purchased there (table 9.1). California requires restaurant chains with 20 or more locations to post calorie information on their menus and indoor menu boards by January 1, 2011. The U.S. Health Care Reform Bill of 2010 also requires chain restaurants and vending machines to post calorie information. Those food companies that are taking an innovative approach in providing lower calorie drinks and smaller portions to help consumers adopt healthier habits may see this labeling as an opportunity to market their more healthful products (Short, 2005). Similarly, others have suggested labeling requirements for soft drink and snack containers sold in movie theaters, convenience stores, and other venues, so that containers have information about calorie, fat, and sugar content. Although there is typically public support for menu labeling, it is unclear what effect it will have, with some early research suggesting no change in dietary choices (Harnack et al., 2008; O'Dougherty et al., 2006). It is difficult to speculate whether consumers simply don't understand dietary guidelines in order to make an appropriate calorie and nutrition choice. It's also possible they don't care, or that other factors, like the perceived value of a larger size at a lower price, are driving dietary choices. It is probably a combination of factors, suggesting that policies may have a better effect when combined with factors at multiple levels, including appropriate consumer education.

As both consumers and food marketing agencies have grown more savvy, additional food labeling expressions, such as *low calorie, few calories, contains a*

TABLE 9.1 Calorie and Fat Content in Selected Fast Foods

Item	Calories	Total fat (g)
Quarter pounder	410	19
Filet-O-Fish	380	18
Medium french fries	380	19
Chicken nuggets (6 pc.)	280	17
Premium Caesar salad w/grilled chicken	220	6
Fruit 'n' yogurt parfait	160	2
Large cola	310	0
Egg McMuffin	300	12

Data from McDonald's USA Nutrition Facts for Popular Menu Items. [Online]. Available: http://nutrition.mcdonalds.com/nutritionexchange/nutritionfacts.pdf [October 6, 2010].

small amount of calories, low source of calories, or *low in calories,* have emerged on food labels. These specific terms are regulated in the United States by the Food and Drug Administration so that consumers can be assured that label claims do indicate that, under very specific circumstances, a food is indeed low in calories, with fewer than 40 calories in 2 tablespoons or 30 grams, depending on the reference amount. The FDA also regulates the terms *low fat, low in fat, contains a small amount of fat, low source of fat,* or *little fat* to indicate that a food has fewer than 3 grams of fat in 2 tablespoons or 30 grams, depending on the reference amount. These kinds of guidelines are helpful for people who are trying to consume fewer calories and less fat; however, a downside to relying on these labels is that they don't offer any information about other important nutritional information. For example, a product may be very low in fat, but very high in added sugars and salts (typically to improve taste in the absence of fat), which may actually contribute to obesity if consumed (USDHHS & USFDA, 2009).

Product price influences consumer purchase and consumption, and the monetary cost of a product is influenced by the costs associated with growing and producing the food. Price represents not only the sticker price but also any discounts and intangible costs, such as transportation, time, attention, or energy involved in purchasing the product. The sticker price can be easily increased through the use of taxes, possibly creating some consumer aversion to the product. Some municipalities have implemented a "sin tax" that taxes foods high in calories and low in nutrients. A recent national survey found that 45% of adults would support a one-cent tax on a can of soft drink, a pound of potato chips, or a pound of butter if the revenues funded a national health education program (Nestle & Jacobson, 2000).

The sticker price is also, in part, driven by agricultural policies. For example, inexpensive candies and other sweet products use corn-based sweetener because it is much cheaper to use corn-based sweetener over sugarcane-based sweetener. This reality is largely driven by heavy U.S. government subsidies to corn growers. Agricultural policies are discussed in more detail in chapter 10. In the United States, it is much less expensive to produce foods high in sugar and fat content as compared to more nutritionally dense foods because these ingredients are cheaper. As a result, foods with more calories and fewer nutrients (e.g., french fries) often cost considerably less than foods with fewer calories and more nutrients (e.g., mixed green salad). Bring low cost together with the high convenience of ready-to-eat foods that are available right through the window of the car, and it is easy to see how price can influence people to rely on diets that promote obesity.

Regulations at the point of purchase also include the promotion of products and all of the marketing of products towards individuals. At the point of purchase, signs, prizes, and incentives can be regulated to enhance or reduce trial and purchase of the product. Despite the potential to regulate promotion, this is probably the least regulated of the four Ps (product, pricing, promotion, and placement) influencing consumer behavior at the point of purchase. The four Ps are discussed further in chapter 13. However, marketing and advertising in other venues is ripe for regulation. Convenience food, fast food, and sugary food make up over 80% of the foods advertised during television programming developed for children. About 44% of the advertising is for candy, sweets, and soft drinks with another 34% for fast foods. In addition, recent data suggest that foods eaten during snack time are depicted more often than foods eaten at breakfast, lunch, and dinner combined (Harrison & Marske, 2005). Scholars and concerned citizens have suggested that television advertising be better regulated to reduce exposure to food advertising, or to mandate equal time for lower calorie, high-nutrient foods. These types of efforts and other regulations at the point of purchase are needed to reduce exposure to obesity-promoting behaviors and increase exposure to health-promoting behaviors.

Incentives for Good Behavior

When asked in interviews, "How would you get people to exercise more?" residents in an urban community answered wholeheartedly, "Pay them!" (Eugeni, Baxter, Mama, & Lee, 2010). Promoting good behavior through incentives can be controversial, but it is a widely used technique in worksites, schools, and even by the government. The key to getting incentives to work is providing an incentive that is strong enough to reinforce the desired behavior.

Worksite wellness policies and programs often include incentives for people to be physically active and maintain a healthy body weight. For example, businesses have tried competitions among employees, in which the person who loses the greatest percentage of body weight wins a prize. Companies may offer monetary incentives for people who commute using active transportation rather than private automobiles, and others give discounts on the worker portion of company insurance premiums for both maintaining a healthy weight and being regularly physically active. Worksite wellness programs are popular among businesses because they improve productivity and morale and reduce sick days, so it is no surprise that worksite fitness objectives from Healthy People 2010 were among the few objectives that have been met (Healthy People 2010, 2009). However, the absence of clear national plans for worksite physical activity may hinder progress in this area in the United States; most of the strategies and tactics of the U.S. National Physical Activity Plan are fairly vague, offering no clear milestones for businesses (U.S. National Physical Activity Plan, 2010). In addition, the long-term effect of worksite incentive programs aimed at increasing physical activity and maintaining healthy weight have not been evaluated.

Other recent regulations have focused on providing tax incentives or credits for weight loss efforts. For example, some have suggested that sales tax be eliminated for the purchase of home exercise equipment, or that employers should be offered incentives to provide weight management programs for their employees. Government agencies could lead this effort by promoting healthy eating in government cafeterias, Veterans Administration medical centers, military installations, prisons, and other venues.

One recent tax credit focused on those who had a diagnosis for an obesity-related, health-compromising condition. Medical expenses paid to lose weight, if it is a treatment for a specific disease that has been diagnosed by a physician, can be deducted. For instance, those taxpayers could deduct costs for joining a weight-loss group and attending regular meetings but not the costs of a spa, health club, or gym; fees for specific weight-loss programs in such facilities are deductible (Internal Revenue Service [IRS], 2009). However, weight-loss expenses for the goal of general good health, appearance, or sense of well-being are not allowable expenses. Special foods could also be deducted if their need was substantiated by a physician (IRS, 2009).

Other Approaches

Many other policy approaches to regulate obesity focused on the individual have been suggested and tried with mixed success. In most cases, policies are not well evaluated in advance, so their efficacy is not determined until after implementation. For example, food assistance programs are widely believed to promote obesity because they rely on a high volume of low-cost foods; however, there is little evidence to support this claim, despite fears. Regardless, it has been suggested that food assistance programs need to be restructured to provide incentives to purchase fruits, vegetables, whole grains, and other nutritionally dense foods (United States Government Accountability Office, 2008).

Educators have also called for medical education to have stronger requirements to teach medical, nursing, and other health professionals the principles and benefits of healthful diet and exercise patterns. Such programs would require health care providers to learn about behavioral risks for obesity and how to counsel patients about health-promoting behavior change, rather than merely diagnosing the disease after the fact. Requirements would need to be supported by a health care system that offered incentives for prevention. For example, Medicaid and Medicare regulations might provide incentives to health care providers for nutrition and obesity counseling and other interventions that meet specified standards of cost and effectiveness.

❏ Understand the background, history, and rationale for policy approaches to improving individual physical activity and eating choices.

❏ Describe how educational policies influence physical activity and dietary habits.

❏ Understand how policies can affect each of the levels of prevention.

❏ Recognize the value of using incentives to encourage healthful behaviors.

Summary

Policies can be powerful determinants of individual behavioral choices that promote or reduce obesity. Policies operate as a set of rules that govern individual behavioral choices and can operate at multiple levels of prevention. The levels of prevention suggest that strategies are needed that address primary, secondary, and tertiary prevention, and that these efforts should be coordinated for maximum impact. Educational approaches provide guidelines for healthful behavior and wellness and are often instituted by governmental agencies. Other educational approaches that affect individual choices involve labeling and pricing strategies to help consumers choose more healthful foods. Incentivizing strategies, such as rewarding healthful behavioral choices, show some popularity and promise for improving healthful choices, particularly at worksites; however, the long-term results of these strategies, as well as most policies, are difficult to identify and remain unknown.

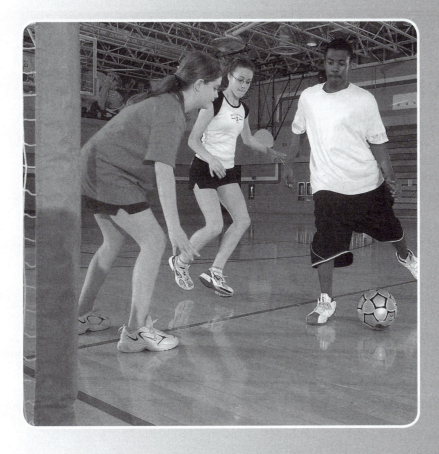

CHAPTER 10

Policy and the Obesogenic Environment

Humans have a long history of policy and regulation with the goals of improving health and behavior. For example, ancient civilizations used policies to regulate allocation of waterways to provide water to residents in nearby municipalities. The use of the water may have been taxed by the government of the day in order to provide capital for the construction of dams or channels to bring the water from the source to the people. These regulations changed the environment by moving the water source closer to the people who needed it and making life possible in areas relatively distant from the original water source. In this book, policies are broadly divided into policies that affect individual knowledge and behavior directly (chapter 9) and policies that influence and change environments themselves, leading to changes in individual behavior. This chapter is not exhaustive in scope but rather highlights policies that have changed the food and physical activity environment.

When we look at the ecologic model (Lee & Cubbin, 2009; Spence & Lee, 2003), we see there are many potential microenvironments that may be affected by policies. For example, schools, worksites, restaurants, physical activity resources, stores, and even personal homes are all governed by policies that change the environment itself. Policies also influence the larger macroenvironment, like national-level trade policies, agricultural regulations, and transportation networks. Policies work at multiple levels, and as a result can sometimes have unexpected consequences—both good and bad. For example, polices aimed at improving roadways for automobiles may have the unintended consequence of making them less hospitable for pedestrians. It is often difficult to predict the unexpected consequences of policies, and sometimes policies will have little impact at all.

Policies usually arise as a result of some identified problem or question that is affecting the public good. For example, trade policies often arise because there is a surplus of desired commodities in one country and a deficit of these same commodities in another country. Moving the commodities from one country to another involves transportation, tariffs, safety, and other logistical factors that all might be easily managed with one good policy. This one good policy can be created and enforced to cover multiple concerns, rather than having to consider each of these individual factors every time the commodity needs to be moved from one country to the other. The consideration of all of these factors is important in policy formulation. A good

Why are policies that regulate the environment potentially more effective than policies that change individual behavior?

policy considers as many factors as possible, including future potential unexpected consequences, and has broad-based support from all constituencies. This support is important to ensure policy adoption by all parties once the policy is implemented.

Policies are adopted by formal agreements and documented for all to review. Once the policy is implemented, it is important to evaluate its efficacy in order to determine if policy modification is needed. Evaluation of policies can be done by third party entities that consider all of the consequences of the policy from an impartial perspective. Formal changes of policies are often made by judicial panels (i.e., the courts) and changed by legislative bodies. This chapter highlights specific policies that have affected or could affect the food and physical activity environment in the promotion or prevention of obesity.

Agriculture

Agricultural policies cover a variety of products and affect consumers by regulating the available food supply. Relevant agricultural policies include farm subsidies, trade embargos, import taxes, farm-to-market incentives, zoning laws regulating rural land use, and food classification and categorization (such as the organic label). Policies that promote healthy food resources are believed necessary to ensure the health of the nation. Changing agriculture to promote healthy food sources has significant implications in terms of economic impact since farming is the second largest component of the U.S. economy (Weber & Becker, 2006). The Farm Security and Rural Investment Act of 2002 consists of 10 components and has an effect on the agriculture and the nutritional value of available foods (USDA, 2002). Farm subsidies under the Farm Bill go mainly to corn, soybeans, wheat, and rice. These foods are important staples in the food supply and also make up a large majority of food ingredients.

In the United States, farm subsidies aimed at corn, soybeans, wheat, and rice were originally enacted to stimulate production of these crops, even in times of economic uncertainty. Producing these crops ensured that both the human and livestock populations would continue to be fed, reducing risk for food insecurity. These policies have worked very well to keep Americans fed and have helped keep the residents of many other countries fed as well via exports to those countries. However, critics have speculated that these policies unwittingly have contributed to the obesity epidemic (Ploeq, 2006). The consistently high production of corn, in particular, contributes to a ready and cheap supply of corn-based sweeteners and fat. Many processed foods use these low-cost, corn-based products, resulting in energy-dense, inexpensive foods available for wide distribution in the marketplace.

High fructose corn syrup and partially hydrogenated corn oil are both blamed for contributing to obesity; however, agricultural policies may be the true culprit underlying reliance on these foods. Favoring these particular foods via incentivizing policies subsequently affects the well-being of the American and global public. The overabundance of high fructose corn syrup is seen in many inexpensive foods like soda and sweet snacks. These can be produced very cheaply, in part because of the use of the very cheap sweeteners. Some believe that this has driven consumption of soda and sweet snacks to an all-time high, despite consistent dietary guidelines favoring higher fruit and vegetable consumption. Some scholars have called for changes in agricultural policies to favor more fruit and vegetable growth in an effort to influence the food supply to favor consumption of fruits and vegetables over cheaply produced, energy-dense snacks (Nestle & Jacobson, 2000).

International Trade

Many policies regulate trade between countries and regions. Policies regulating trade are formed with the food supply in mind, but they also may reflect geography and political alliances. For example, goals of strengthening the political alliance between the United States and China have led to increases in food imports from China to the United States, along with increases in trade in noncomestibles. Increases in trade improve the variety of available foods, potentially leading to greater nutritional opportunity but also potentially contributing to obesity. Many have blamed the export of American fast food as a primary contributor to the obesity epidemic in countries outside of the United States. In reality, it is difficult to say who is to blame. The introduction of very energy-dense foods has increased demand for them, so now many countries offer their own local versions of fried, energy-dense, nutritionally poor food, potentially a greater contributor to obesity than imported food.

Food Industry and Food Environments

Just as many agricultural policies are aimed at improving the quality of the food supply, the food industry also must adhere to regulations that protect consumers from poor quality or unsafe foods. The food industry is required to use food labels to inform the public concerning the ingredients in food. Because the food industry often has a relatively large profit margin, many policy makers have advocated for stronger polices to help guide the food industry. For example, food makers can provide a broader range of products to appeal to both good health and good taste, improving the food environment for consumers. The motivation for the food industry to change is related to economic impact; that is, if companies have healthier products, they may be able to sell them to a larger market share. Thus there is an advantage to exploring and producing alternative food products.

For food policy to be sustainable and accepted, partnerships with food and beverage industries are necessary. Although public health policy may create an emphasis on cooperative consumer and corporation partnerships, there is a need for policies and legislation that regulate the activities of corporations. Other strategies have included social pressure and legal action against companies that produce less healthy products and enacting policies to manage advertisement and marketing (Nestle & Jacobson, 2000). Regulating advertisements or increasing taxes on junk food does not reduce the number of choices for the individual but rather changes the food environment. Food advertisement is a ubiquitous element in the food environment (discussed in chapters 13 and 14). Regulations on advertising have reduced advertisement of alcohol and tobacco products, which in turn, has led to changes in consumer behavior. Consumers tend to desire products that are more heavily advertised. Regulations to reduce the advertising of energy-dense foods might also result in less interest from consumers. In contrast, policies to stimulate marketing of healthful foods like fresh fruits and vegetables might increase interest in these products from consumers.

Product regulations concern the actual ingredients of the product; these ingredients are regulated by the U.S. Food and Drug Administration to ensure that they are safe for human consumption. Recent efforts have begun to regulate trans-fatty acids in foods. Trans-fatty acids are partially hydrogenated vegetable oils that have been modified to have a shelf life longer than traditional shortenings used in baked goods and a better ability to withstand higher temperatures for longer periods of time than traditional oils used in restaurant fryers. Several American cities have enacted bans on trans-fatty acids in response to consumer concerns about the safety of trans fat. These bans have changed the food environment, making it impossible for consumers to choose trans fat. This kind of policy improves the quality of the food environment directly and improves the quality of the dietary habits of consumers indirectly.

Product regulations may also extend to the size or number of portions in the product being sold. For example, the practice of supersizing leads to product packaging with multiple portions in a single package, encouraging over consumption. Government recommendations for portion sizes are often based on relatively modest portions, and consumers may not always realize that the product that they are consuming represents multiple portions. Some scholars have called for an end to the practice of supersizing, deeming it unfair to consumers who may be duped into believing that they are consuming less than they actually are. In contrast, other companies have responded to the millions of Americans who demand single-serving packaging, such as 100-calorie packs and smaller bottles and cans of soft drinks and juices. Standardizing serving sizes would change the food environment, reducing the available options of portion sizes; it might also assist consumers to control dietary intake more effectively.

Placement of stores and restaurants in neighborhoods may contribute to dietary habits and obesity among residents. Many major store and restaurant chains endeavor to place their stores in particular neighborhoods based on demographic factors. Zoning policies can regulate where stores are allowed to be built; for example, regulations may prohibit fast-food or convenience stores from opening near schools to reduce the probability that children will visit them to buy high-calorie foods. Geographic epidemiologic analyses have found that many low socioeconomic areas often contain many more fast-food restaurants and convenience stores as compared to high socioeconomic areas (Adams et al., 2002; Chung, 1999; Moore & Diez Roux, 2006; Sooman,

Macintyre, & Anderson, 1993; Wang, Kim, Gonzalez, MacLeod, & Winkleby, 2007; Zenk et al., 2005). These environments can promote unhealthy eating habits in populations that are already at an increased risk for overweight and obesity.

Policies can also influence where the food is placed in stores. Food producers ideally would like food products at the eye level of the target consumer to stimulate trial and purchase of the product. For example, foods that are marketed to children may be placed at the child's eye level, not the parent's. Regulations could be implemented to reduce children seeing and asking for particular foods by raising the level at which they are displayed. Other placement regulations have called for a requirement that venders provide equal shelf space for high-calorie, low-nutrient foods and low-calorie, high-nutrient foods; however, few communities have adopted such policies.

Another set of policies about food placement in recent history concerns vending machines. In the United States, there are over 3 million vending machines located in schools, parks, and nearly everywhere else (American Council for an Energy Efficient Economy, 2009). One soda maker stated, "To build pervasiveness of our products, we're putting ice-cold Coca-Cola classic and our other brands within reach, wherever you look: at the supermarket, the video stores, the soccer field, the gas station—everywhere" (Coca-Cola Company, 2007). Placement of vending machines has become an especially big concern for schools, who receive money from the company for allowing the machine to be placed in the school, and who may receive some of the profits from the machine. The Los Angeles Unified School District banned vending machines in schools because of the deep concern that such ready access to sugared drinks might promote obesity (Hayasaki, 2002). Banning vending machines has since become a widespread strategy, and many cities have sought to reduce such easy access to convenience foods, reflecting a change in the food environment. Concerns about child health have led to policies that been adopted or are under consideration by many U.S. states. For example, the Texas Public School Nutrition Policy was implemented to limit the availability of foods with very low nutritional quality; reduce or ban fried foods, particularly french fries and competitive foods; and increase fruit, vegetable, and reduced-fat milk availability (Department of Agriculture, 2010). This policy has demonstrated improvements in the dietary quality of youth at school, increasing fruit, vegetable, and milk consumption and decreasing consumption of less desirable foods (sweetened beverages, fried foods) (Cullen, Watson, & Zakeri, 2008; Mendoza, Watson, & Cullen, 2010).

Built Environment

Regulating the built environment has been gaining in popularity since studies have determined that neighborhood design and structures can contribute to healthy lifestyles. Often, zoning laws will determine what kinds of structures can be built in a neighborhood. The state of North Carolina noted that there are many complex environmental determinants of obesity and, in 2006, took steps towards obesity reduction ("Eat Smart Move More," 2006). The state encouraged focus on a dynamic plan to reduce obesity by increasing awareness of health promotion behaviors related to physical activity and healthy diet. This plan included statewide initiatives, policies, and funding to promote healthy eating, as well as physical activity infrastructure, such as parks and community centers, that promotes physical activity. All were believed necessary efforts to change the obesogenic nature of neighborhoods.

Many neighborhoods have recently begun to focus on smart growth using new principles of urbanism for development. Smart growth offers residents a range of housing options, from single family homes to apartments; and emphasizes neighborhood features that foster walkability over drivability as well as mixed-use development, where homes are located near schools, goods, and services. This is a departure from the suburban developments that have dominated neighborhood development in the United States for the past 50 years. This trend has been driven by scientific findings suggesting that more compact neighborhoods with mixed-use development have higher rates of physical activity and lower rates of obesity (discussed in greater detail in chapter 4 on the built environment). This type of neighborhood development is also favored by many consumers who prefer a greater sense of community with neighbors.

Local governments have realized that smart growth is advantageous economically and environmentally. Policies have begun to allocate funding for smart growth development, including elements that foster active transportation, such as bikeways and protected pedestrian pathways. In existing developments, agencies have begun to provide guides for cities, zoning authorities, and urban planners; these guides suggest ways to modify zoning requirements, designate downtown areas as pedestrian malls and automobile-free zones, and modify residential neighborhoods, workplaces, and shopping centers to promote physical activity. These guides and strategies have been distributed and implemented in the hope of reducing obesity in the population. More innovative municipalities have begun to provide funding for multiuse recreation centers and parks, particularly in low-income neighborhoods. As of 2009, the California Office of Grants and Local Services was administering grant programs that provide funds to local and state agencies and other organizations for park, recreation, and resource-related projects. Another organization in California, the Marin Community Foundation, provides community grants for access to parks and open spaces. It supports projects that increase the access that low-income and minority individuals have to parks (Marin Community Foundation, 2009).

Along with promoting active transportation, many municipalities have begun to develop their public transportation and bicycling infrastructure, recognizing that this reduces the environmental burden of personal automobiles.

Implementing Policy

Congestion Road Tax

Policies aimed at improving quality of life in one domain often have additional consequences in other domains. Stockholm, Sweden implemented a congestion road tax, with the hope that by taxing all major roads in and out of Stockholm, both automobile and air traffic would be reduced. At the same time, it was hoped that there would be increased use of public transportation. Regular use of public transportation is reliably associated with increases in physical activity, in part driven by the simple act of walking or biking to and from the transit stops. Electronic sensors scanned pictures of license plates and recorded car trips, and the system sent drivers a bill once a month. The congestion road tax increased moderate intensity physical activity and decreased the time spent sitting down. By making driving more costly and less desirable than other commuting strategies via financial disincentives, the city was able to reduce traffic congestion, improve air quality, and increase physical activity among those who would normally commute by automobile (Bergman, Grjibovski, Hagstromer, Patterson, & Sjostrom, 2010; Besser & Dannenberg, 2005).

Although this policy is not targeting obesity specifically, communities with better public transportation opportunities and bicycling and pedestrian infrastructure tend to have residents that use alternative transportation. Those residents tend to get more daily physical activity compared to residents of neighborhoods with poor public transportation opportunities and poor active transportation infrastructure, reducing, in part, the public health burden of obesity in the community (Besser & Dannenberg, 2005; Wen & Rissel, 2008). For example, California passed the Complete Streets Act of 2007, mandating that cities and counties ensure that the circulation element of the general plan addresses the needs of pedestrians, bicyclists, and transit riders (figure 10.1) (National Complete Streets Coalition, 2007).

Transportation

The transportation network in a community represents the infrastructure available to support transportation opportunities for residents. Transportation regulations can foster environments that are more or less suitable for active transportation (described in greater detail in chapter 6). For example, neighborhoods that offer well-maintained sidewalks, attractive routes, a variety of routes, and protected pedestrian pathways and bikeways present a better infrastructure for active transportation than neighborhoods that have large streets with higher traffic volume. Many cities in Asia, Australia, Europe, and

Why do we need Complete Streets policies?

Complete Streets improve safety.

A Federal Highways Administration safety review found that streets designed with sidewalks, raised medians, better bus stop placement, traffic-calming measures, and treatments for disabled travelers improve pedestrian safety. Some features, such as medians, improve safety for all users: they enable pedestrians to cross busy roads in two stages, reduce left-turning motorist crashes to zero, and improve bicycle safety.

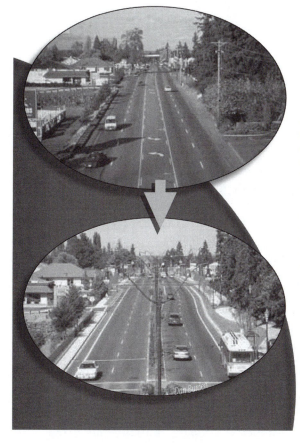

Complete Streets encourage walking and bicycling for health.

The National Institutes of Medicine recommends fighting childhood obesity by establishing ordinances to encourage construction of sidewalks, bikeways, and other places for physical activity. A recent study funded by the National Institutes of Health found those who lived in walkable neighborhoods got 30 to 45 minutes more exercise each week than those living in low-walkable areas. Residents of walkable communities were also less likely to be overweight or obese.

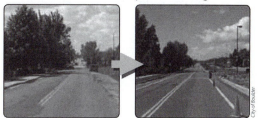

Complete Streets address climate change and oil dependence.

The potential to reduce carbon emissions by shifting trips to lower-carbon modes is undeniable. The 2001 National Household Transportation Survey found 50% of all trips in metropolitan areas are three miles or less and 28% of all metropolitan trips are one mile or less – distances easy to walk, bike, or hop a bus or train. Yet 65% of the shortest trips are now made by automobile, in part because of incomplete streets that make it dangerous or unpleasant for other modes of travel. Complete streets would help convert many of these short automobile trips to multi-modal travel. Simply increasing bicycling from 1% to 1.5% of all trips in the U.S. would save 462 million gallons of gasoline each year. Using transit has already helped the United States save 1.5 billion gallons of fuel each year since the early 1990s, which is nearly 36 million barrels of oil.

Complete Streets foster strong communities.

Complete streets play an important role in livable communities, where all people – regardless of age, ability or mode of transportation – feel safe and welcome on the roadways. A safe walking and bicycling environment is an essential part of improving public transportation and creating friendly, walkable communities.

FIGURE 10.1 This section of a Complete Streets brochure provides information on complete streets.

Courtesy of National Complete Streets Coalition.

North America have implemented bicycle sharing systems, where a fleet of bicycles is available for use by the public for short-distance travel and commuting. Citizens have to register and pay in advance or per use, borrowing and returning the bicycle to a specific location (DeMaio, 2008; Pucher, Dill, & Handy, 2010). Although considerable investment is required by a municipality to supply and maintain the bicycles and bikeways and administer the programs, coordinated municipal bike share programs are effective for increasing travel by bicycle and thereby increasing physical activity.

Regulations and policies to improve the environment for active transportation arise during municipal development and often come into play again during redevelopment and renewal activities. Sometimes policies that govern automobiles affect the transportation environment as well. For example, lower speed limits for automobiles, a policy that may be aimed at conserving fuel, may have the additional benefit of improving the safety of roadways for cyclists and pedestrians. Slower automobiles are easier to control than faster automobiles. This is the argument behind policies that reduce the speed of automobiles on roads close to schools, potentially improving the safety of the physical activity environment for children who are attending the school.

The initial design of communities with a variety of transportation options is important for fostering multi-use transportation environments. Although the move toward new urbanism has improved many policies aimed at active transportation, there are still areas that could be improved. Policies are needed to provide ongoing support to communities. As time goes by, roads, sidewalks, and other elements of the transportation environment, like amenities such as lighting, water fountains, and trees, need to be maintained. Funds to support maintenance are typically allocated from local municipal budgets; thus, policies to maintain these budget allocations are very important (Lopez & Hynes, 2006).

Another important element in the transportation environment is public transportation. Reliance on public transportation is associated with higher rates of physical activity and lower rates of obesity (Bell, Ge, & Popkin, 2002; Wen & Rissel, 2008). Many people in newer, westernized countries prefer to drive personal automobiles rather than take public transportation. In order for public transportation to be a fully functional and important part of the environment, it must be made easier, more pleasant, more convenient, and more cost effective compared to driving a personal automobile.

Schools

Many policies have been enacted in the education system, with the bulk of the education policy having to do with food and physical activity opportunities that are available during the school day. Information distributed in schools has the potential to affect nearly all children who attend school regularly. More than 95% of American children from ages 5 to 17 are enrolled in school

(Story, Kaphingst, & French, 2006). Children are in school for at least 180 days a year, suggesting that food available at the school may represent a sizable portion of the meals eaten by the average child in America.

The long-overdue U.S. Child Nutrition and WIC Reauthorization Act was signed into law in 2004 to build on the original 1966 Child Nutrition Act that provided healthful food during the school day. The 2004 Child Nutrition Act sought to include nutrition and physical education and updated food standards in American schools. It requires schools to define nutrition guidelines for all food sold during the school day and set goals for nutrition education and physical activity. The 2004 Child Nutrition Act also requires local wellness policies to be developed and implemented by parents, teachers, administrators, school food service, school boards, and the public to provide better coordination between schools and other individuals and organizations who may provide care and service for children (USDA Food and Nutrition Service, 2004). California, for example, passed an act in 2008 to ensure that schools were complying with nutritional standards for the sale of á la carte and vending machine items.

School meal programs have gained more attention in terms of healthy selections and have significantly improved over the past 15 years with the onset of the Dietary Guidelines for Americans. The 2004 Child Nutrition Act helped to revise regulations for school lunches and requires that cow's milk be provided daily. Although this regulation was a long time coming, the next steps for this kind of regulation would be to require that any foods that compete with school meals be consistent with federal recommendations for fat, saturated fat, cholesterol, sugar, and sodium content. More recent evaluation and guidelines for school lunches have suggested that most schools are severely lacking in their lunchtime offerings, with over-reliance on fried foods and sodium with lower nutritional density and little variety (Stallings, Suitor, & Taylor, 2010). Public school lunches have been typically underfunded, so schools have been limited in the quality of food that could be provided. Other efforts may be needed to enhance funding for schools to meet these guidelines and improve the health of children.

In terms of enhancing the physical activity environment among schools, funding could be allocated to schools via policy efforts to help enhance and fund daily physical education and sports programs in primary and secondary schools, extending the school day if necessary. Other school-based strategies to promote health and prevent obesity might focus on banning soda and nutritionally vacuous snacks. Many schools also rely on television programming in the classrooms that exposes students to commercials for foods high in calories, fat, or sugar on school television programs (for example, Channel One). Policies could incentivize schools that do not expose children to this kind of potentially harmful marketing. Many of these more specialized and costly policy fixes may occur at the local level, rather than at a state or federal level.

Worksites

The worksite environment has also been the focus of policy. Broad calls for multilevel worksite wellness strategies have underscored the importance of supportive worksite environments (American Heart Association, 2009; Katz et al., 2005). In the United States, 65% of the population over the age of 16 works in traditional worksite settings, making the worksite an ideal place to reach adults (Clark, Iceland, Palumbo, Posey, & Weismantle, 2003). A recent study published in 2009 suggests that until 2006, in the United States, only a few states (e.g., North Dakota, Oklahoma, Washington) have enacted legislative bills aimed at worker wellness policies (Lankford, Kruger, & Bauer, 2009). It may be more likely that smaller scale, worksite-specific, microenvironmental policies may regulate what can be offered in work cafeterias or the kind of physical activity settings that are available at the worksite. For example, work cafeterias may change their plate or container sizes, influencing portion sizes that are available. Another strategy implemented by some worksites might involve the ingredients in the food. Food can be prepared using ingredients lower in calories derived from unnecessary fat or additional sugar (Pratt et al., 2007). Improving the available food supply could be coupled with allowing healthy weight management groups to hold meetings during lunch or after hours.

Employers also may invest in fitness, grooming, and locker facilities and allow flexible schedules with time to do physical activity during the workday (Phipps, Madison, Pomerantz, & Klein, 2010; Pratt et al., 2007). In place of coffee or smoking breaks, physical activity breaks involving stretches, short bursts of cardio activity, yoga, or tai-chi could be implemented to help provide interesting opportunities in the work setting. Short physical activity breaks can transform workplace culture. Management that supports and encourages physical activity in a work day so that groups of coworkers can regularly participate in physical activity breaks enhances social support and enjoyment during the work day (Taylor, 2005).

In a bid to reduce traffic congestion, the U.S. state of Washington enacted the Commute Trip Reduction Tax Credit, requiring major employers in large counties to implement commute trip reduction programs ("Commute Trip Reduction Tax Credit," 2005). Employers received tax credits for providing financial incentives to employees who share rides or use public transit or active transportation. Although this type of policy has great benefit for the environment, it also holds promise to increase physical activity directly by increasing active transportation and indirectly by improving the physical activity environment through reduced air pollution and improved street safety with fewer cars. To date, no research has been done to evaluate the health effects of this policy.

Regardless of the strategy, it is clear that changing the worksite environment is an important part of obesity prevention and control (Aldana, 2001; Chapman, 2005). Worksite wellness programs have been shown to significantly reduce sick days and improve worker productivity. It's no wonder: People with access to worksite services such as fitness counseling, gyms, and equipment are approximately two times more likely to meet daily physical activity goals (Dodson, Lovegreen, Elliott, Haire-Joshu, & Brownson, 2008). Worksite policies incorporating infrastructure that supports improved access to resources may have a greater chance of success (Kahn et al., 2002; Matson-Koffman, Brownstein, Neiner, & Greaney, 2005). When employees are in health-promoting environments for most of their waking hours, it is likely that this exposure will affect home and family life as well. Thus, there are many benefits to be gained from simple changes in worksite policies that reduce the obesogenic capacity of the worksite.

❏ Understand how policies that directly change the environment can indirectly change individual behavioral choices and reduce or prevent obesity.

❏ Describe the divergent effects of agricultural policies that improve the food supply but might contribute to obesity.

❏ Identify policies that influence the built environment and transportation to improve the physical activity environment.

❏ Describe the strategy and effects of policies that change school and work environments to foster physical activity and improved dietary habits.

GETTING STARTED

Summary

Policies targeting the obesogenic environment can be quite complex but when executed with careful planning and enforcement, they can improve the greater good while not over-regulating or burdening any one person or procedure. Policies that influence the obesogenic environment are varied, and they function in agriculture, trade, marketing, transportation, school, and worksite settings. It may be argued that the policies that improve the quality of the environment are the most foolproof because the available behavioral choices that humans can make are health promoting. For example, many people may have a much harder time choosing fresh fruit, a green salad, or steamed vegetables if there are french fries available. However, if the only options in the food environment are healthful, then it is easier to select a healthful choice. Policies that affect the individual directly may be less sustainable because the choice to misbehave may be too challenging. More could be done to capitalize on the universal benefit that policies may bring to enhance health; however, policies must be supported by a broad constituency in order to be sustainable. As well, policies are dynamic, just like humans and environments are, so it is important to evaluate and re-evaluate their impact and consequences. When policies do more harm than good, it is important to revise them and continue the process.

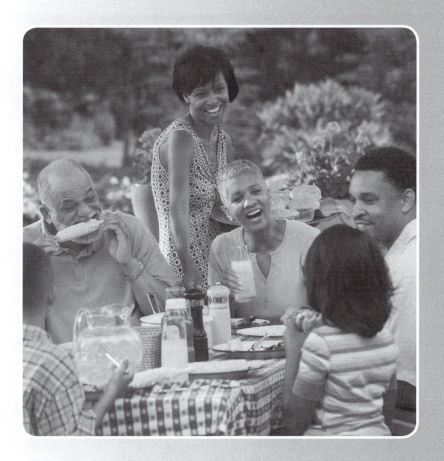

CHAPTER 11

Cultural
and Familial Influences

As scientists and clinicians attempt to investigate and treat the obesity epidemic, cultural and familial influences on physical activity, dietary habits, and obesity have emerged as significant influences on individual health. Ecologic models suggest that various environmental factors affect health behavior, which can, in turn, lead to obesity (Spence & Lee, 2003). In particular, social environments, like culture and family, have evolved into complex and multifaceted determinants of health outcomes.

Cultural diversity affects health perspectives and health behaviors. Culture refers to practices and rituals that are conveyed or inherited via family and cultural institutions. It does not include socioeconomic factors like income, occupation, or place of residence, but it may include things like eating patterns, music preferences, and religious beliefs (Sankofa & Johnson-Taylor, 2007). Different cultures may have diverse cultural practices that include various definitions of health and attractiveness, assumptions related to causes of illness, and curative strategies like indigenous healers or remedies. Last, cultural traditions affect food selection and preparation (Airhihenbuwa et al., 1996).

Race and ethnicity refer to classifications of people based on genetic and phenotypical characteristics, family origin, and historical and political preferences. Race is a relatively arbitrary classification that is typically based on physical features such as skin pigmentation and facial and hair characteristics. Racial classification dates back to ancient times and historically referred to three races, African or Negroid, Asian or Mongoloid, and European or Caucasoid. In recent history, the terms black, Asian, and white have increased in use over the more archaic definitions. Racial classification is used in the United States along with many other countries for official classification of citizens, but even this is not consistent. Racial identity and classification has been socially and politically controversial at times and tends to be too broad a classification for much use with regard to health behaviors and outcomes.

Ethnicity is somewhat more useful because it is more directly based on a person's family origins. *Hispanic* is typically considered an ethnic category, and people of Hispanic ethnicity may be black, brown, white, or mixed, and even Asian. Within ethnic categories there are often many unique cultures, and globalization has produced many individuals who draw on a plurality of cultures. It is helpful to consider ethnicity and culture together as they provide a more distinct and true representation of factors that might affect physical activity, dietary habits, and obesity.

Family and Culture Within the Ecologic Model of Obesity

As described in earlier chapters, ecologic models include multiple levels, such as macro-, exo-, meso-, and microenvironmental dimensions, and can encompass familial and cultural factors (Egger & Swinburn, 1997; Lee & Cubbin, 2002; Spence & Lee, 2003). The microsystem is composed of the social settings where individuals interact and includes homes, work, parks, and schools. Family roles, preferences, and individual cultures can be embedded within these systems and influence individual and societal health behaviors. For example, when, where, and how an individual is raised can affect one's eating behavior as well as the social environments that the adult chooses to interact in. Familial exchanges and influences (e.g., a child being influenced by parents' eating habits) occur at the microsystem (home) level and can also be associated with the macroenvironment. Earlier studies have provided a close examination of these settings and revealed associations between the environment and obesity prevalence in its encompassing residents (Crossman, Anne Sullivan, & Benin, 2006; Merten, Williams, & Shriver, 2009).

Within the larger obesogenic social environment, cultural practices and beliefs and family responsibilities, roles, and preferences can influence dietary habits, physical activity, and obesity. For example, an individual's culture can influence eating habits like food choices and portion sizes. Even within the same culture, various family health behaviors can deviate from the cultural norm, depending upon outside influences and personal preferences. A child might choose to be a vegetarian while being raised in a home that frequently includes meat as part of the diet. Another example might be a Jewish employee who celebrates Christmas and eats cake and cookies at a Secret Santa office party. These individuals are interacting and engaging in health behaviors that are not necessarily part of their personal culture or family norms.

An individual's culture and family can also influence physical activity. Over time, various cultures have preferred particular sports. Tradition, social experiences, and preferences can be associated with the types and amounts of physical activity someone does (Khanam & Costarelli, 2008). For example, if parents teach a young child how to play baseball, then the child might choose to play baseball at school with friends. The child is familiar with the sport because of family learning experiences, and, in turn, chooses to play at school because of comfort and familiarity with the game. Furthermore, the types of physical activity family members choose can be associated with the choices of any other given family member or the family as a whole (Laskarzewski et al., 1983). In our baseball example, perhaps the child's younger sibling witnesses the family playing baseball and wants to participate in the activity as well. This could prompt physical activity in the younger child's life also.

Members of some ethnic groups and families appear more vulnerable to obesity, perhaps driven in part by complex genetic predispositions to obesity. This chapter does not discuss genetic predispositions but focuses only on cultural and familial influences of the obesogenic environment. The associations of culture and family with health behaviors are discussed in relation to the obesogenic environment.

Cultural Influences

Although the United States has always been a melting pot, as obesity has increased dramatically over the past few decades, attention to cultural and familial influences on health behaviors and obesity has also significantly increased. U.S. culture is not a simple, uniform entity that embodies one type of lifestyle; it is a combination of civilizations involving complex and diverse predictors of health. Culture is defined as decisively conveyed and inherited practices that do not include socioeconomic factors like income, occupation, or place of residence, and can be displayed across a variety of domains including, but not limited to, eating patterns, physical activity preferences, and religious beliefs (Sankofa & Johnson-Taylor, 2007). Cultures can vary among different races and ethnicities and can include various traditions, styles, and more.

Acculturation to the majority culture, or the exchange of cultural features that results when groups come into continuous contact, has been associated with diabetes and unhealthy behaviors for some populations (Mainous, Diaz, & Geesey, 2008). Some data also suggest that acculturation into Western culture is associated with overweight and obesity (Popkin & Udry, 1998). Furthermore, diverse international traditions and customs have emerged as important influences of the social obesogenic environment (Spence & Lee, 2003).

Cultural Influences on Dietary Habits

Culture has an important influence on health behaviors and health outcomes. In particular, culture has increasingly influenced the American diet in recent years. The typical American diet largely consists of overprocessed, packaged food that is excessively energy dense (Wells, 2006). For example, fast food has an average energy density 145% greater than that of a traditional African diet (Prentice & Jebb, 2003). A traditional African diet typically includes a combination of locally available fruits, cereal grains, vegetables, milk, and meat products (Eatoutzone, 2007). In a fast-paced, technology-driven society, fast food has become a staple in many Americans' diets, causing various health problems. Culture is associated with food choices, food accessibility, celebrations, and portion sizes. All are important predictors of dietary habits and are discussed below in more detail.

Food choices and preferences differ among cultures and ethnicities. For example, studies of black Americans have suggested consumption of a low level of fruits and vegetables and a high level of high-fat pork products and products containing dietary cholesterol (Kumanyika & Ewart, 1990). In particular, black women tend to have a higher preference for sweet foods and beverages and are sometimes more hesitant to limit dietary fat intake (Kumanyika, 1987). Other data suggest that the dietary habits of Latinos who are less acculturated to U.S. society are healthier than those of Latinos who are more acculturated (Perez-Escamilla & Putnik, 2007).

Food accessibility, along with limited individual economic resources, tends to run along cultural lines. In the United States, as well as other industrialized nations, recent immigrants tend to have fewer economic resources, limiting their options for food. Immigrants may come from a thriving culture in another country but be among a minority group in the new country of residence. Several studies have shown that racial and ethnic minorities and socioeconomically disadvantaged populations have an increased risk of obesity (Ford & Dzewaltowski, 2008; Heinrich et al., 2008). Low SES areas, particularly public housing neighborhoods, typically have fewer grocery stores, less access to fresh produce like fruits and vegetables, and more fast-food restaurants and convenience stores (Lee et al., 2009; Regan, Lee, Booth, & Reese-Smith, 2006). These factors, including limited economic resources, can restrict healthy food options and contribute to an increased risk of obesity within socioeconomically disadvantaged populations (Ford & Dzewaltowski, 2008).

Cultural celebrations also can influence dietary habits. Feasting, the participation in a feast or heartily eating, is a common practice in most cultures. Some cultural celebrations involve the consumption of sugary or high-fat foods like birthday cakes, Halloween candy, Thanksgiving dinners, and feasts celebrating religious events like Eid ul-Fitr and Christmas. These eating rituals can differ depending on one's culture, religion, or belief system. For example, some cultures do not recognize Halloween or Christmas but celebrate other holidays (e.g., Hanukkah, Day of the Dead). These cultural celebrations may or may not include nutritious foods like fruits and vegetables. American holidays, like the Fourth of July, sometimes include grilling hamburgers or other types of red meat. Although cultural celebrations vary, all are important influences on dietary habits.

Despite the vast array of cultures residing in many Westernized nations, overall portion sizes have increased tremendously in the past quarter century, often blamed on American lack of restraint (Nielsen & Popkin, 2003). Some restaurant portion sizes in the United States are now almost three times the standard serving size. Larger, family-serving styles, sometimes popular in Italian, Korean, and other cultures, can also hinder portion control. Furthermore, some cultures that are more historically prone to economic hardships might be more likely to overeat at meals for fear of future famines

> Describe the intergenerational transmission of health habits. Why are these important?

or decreased income (Olson, Bove, & Miller, 2007; Smith & Richards, 2008). For example, some Americans who lived during the Great Depression might be more prone to eat all of the food served (an increased portion size) at a meal out of a fear of food loss or out of a habit of conservation. Often, these cultural beliefs and eating habits are passed intergenerationally, even when food security is no longer a concern.

Changing cultural practices and beliefs regarding dietary habits is needed in order to repair the social elements in the obesogenic environment. Although cultural dietary practices are often systemic and deeply rooted, they can be amended to include healthy foods. Educating individuals and cultural groups about healthier substitutions (e.g., replacing red meat with fish) and celebratory eating practices (e.g., grilling vegetables instead of, or along with, hamburgers) may spark a change within a cultural group or society. Educating parents and children on appropriate portion sizes can stop the intergenerational passing of overfeeding practices and culturally born beliefs of food insecurity.

Cultural Influences on Physical Activity

Culture also has a significant influence on physical activity. People from different cultures prefer different leisure time physical activities and sports. Different cultural factors like social preferences, accessibility of playing, feasibility of learning the physical activity, and the inclusiveness of participants all influence physical activity.

Different cultures favor certain types of physical activity, and some sports and physical activities require more people to participate or more social interaction. For instance, some studies have supported the idea of social support as an important predictor of physical activity for African American women (Richter, Wilcox, Greaney, Henderson, & Ainsworth, 2002; Wilbur, Chandler, Dancy, & Lee, 2003). These data suggest that the more social support these women had, the more likely they were to be physically active.

Many types of physical activity and sports foster social support and social interactions. Sports like football, basketball, and baseball encourage social outings and social engagement. For example, baseball, a socially interactive and popular spectator sport, is more popular than diving, an individual sport. Similarly, soccer, or fútbol, is popular among many Latino cultures. Latino cultures typically value social activities and family relationships.

One's place of residence, a factor often related to culture, can also be a determinant of physical activity. For instance, people of similar cultures often choose to live in similar geographic areas or close to one another, like urban or suburban areas. People living in more confined, urban areas with less green space are further limited in the types of physical activity and sports they can do. For example, people living in New York City are probably less likely to have the green space to play a game of football compared to people living in a suburb of Houston. Furthermore, some cultures reside in physical environments, such as extreme heat or cold, that are not conducive to outside physical activity. For instance, Central Americans and people living in some southern parts of the United States endure extreme heat for several months a year, sometimes deterring physical activity performed outside. These logistical physical activity requirements can often vary by place of residence and culture.

Like dietary habits, cultural influences on physical activity are often deeply rooted and transmitted intergenerationally. Educating individuals and cultural groups on the benefits of physical activity and various forms of physical activity, particularly unfamiliar sports or games, can help to promote and improve levels of physical activity, as can fostering social support and improving the accessibility of physical activity equipment and environments for underserved cultures.

Ethnic and Cultural Influences on Obesity

Not only does culture influence dietary habits and physical activity, specific ethnic groups are significantly more vulnerable to obesity (Flegal, Carroll, Ogden, & Johnson, 2010). Figure 11.1 depicts this trend in obesity prevalence in the United States from 2006-2008. Cultural influences on physical activity and dietary habits that may then contribute to obesity do not necessarily take ethnicity into account, although many cultural health beliefs and practices are based on ethnicity. Using the earlier example of immigration, individuals and groups can be of different ethnicities, migrate to the United States, and acculturate to this nation's dominant culture. This acculturation can lead to new dietary habits, physical activity levels, and often a change of cultural beliefs and perceptions that can lead to obesity. It may be that people who are more recent migrants to a dominant western culture are at higher risk of developing obesity.

Other Cultural Beliefs and Perceptions

Cultural influences on dietary habits, physical activity, and obesity aren't the only cultural influences of the obesogenic environment. Cultural beliefs and perceptions can significantly affect the obesogenic environment. Body

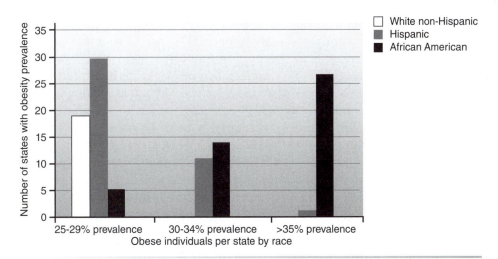

FIGURE 11.1 Obesity prevalence among different ethnic or racial groups in the United States from 2006 to 2008.

Data from Centers for Disease Control and Prevention, 2007, "Differences in prevalence of obesity among black, white, and Hispanic adults—United States, 2006-2008," *Morbidity and Mortality Weekly Report* 58(27): 740-744.

image, attitudes, and physical activity perceptions can promote or deter health behaviors that can lead to an increased risk for obesity.

More relaxed attitudes toward an overweight or obese body image are significant predictors of health behaviors for some cultures and particularly children (Kumanyika, 1993; Pinhey, Rubenstein, & Colfax, 1997). For example, some studies suggest that larger bodies are more valued and less discriminated against among Mississippi Choctaw, American Samoan, and black women as compared to white women (Bindon, Dressler, Gilliland, & Crews, 2007). Black women are less likely to diet for aesthetic reasons or be body-conscious (Bennett, 1991). Perhaps some black women experience less culture-based pressure to diet for the sake of appearance than do white women (Kumanyika, Morssink, & Agurs, 1992). Also, some studies have shown that black men may not consider a woman's weight to be a deterrent when it comes to partnering and may find overweight women more attractive than white men do (Harris, Walters, & Waschull, 1991; Thomas & James, 1988). Adolescent white females are also more likely to perceive themselves as overweight when compared to the self-perceptions of adolescent black females (Neff, Sargent, McKeown, Jackson, & Valois, 1997). These cultural stereotypical body images are often portrayed by the media and can affect body dissatisfaction and food intake (Anschutz, Engels, Becker, & van Strien, 2008). Despite these cultural preferences, most ethnicities tend to acculturate to the American norm over time (Popkin & Udry, 1998).

The rise in childhood obesity has been complicated by beliefs that a chubby baby is a healthy baby. Theorists have suggested that in Asian and Latino cultures, children who are heavier are more likely to survive hardship. In some cases, increasing weight in children may be viewed as an indicator of wealth, suggesting that families have sufficient resources to support children and offspring (Haslam & James, 2005).

In addition, cultural physical activity perceptions are also important predictors of health behaviors and obesity. Some cultures might view exercise as work or a physical struggle. For example, for some blacks in the United States, physical activity is perceived as structured exercise and not as incidental activity of daily life (Tudor-Locke et al., 2003). Furthermore, for low-income populations working long hours, multiple jobs, or both, being physically active might be perceived as additional work (Henderson & Ainsworth, 2003). Perceiving physical activity as additional work is likely to discourage leisure-time physical activity. One problem with this perception and the resulting behavior is that it serves as a sedentary role model to others in the family and community. Even if the originator of these beliefs achieves sufficient levels of physical activity for weight maintenance, a pattern of sedentary living is exhibited to others. This pattern can be intergenerationally transmitted, promoting sedentary lifestyles to offspring, placing them at higher risk for obesity.

Addressing and changing cultural beliefs and practices that contribute to obesity is necessary. Education and mass media efforts may be useful tools for change. For example, media personalities and celebrities often shape cultural beliefs, particularly body image, and can be used as role models to help repair unhealthy perceptions. Other cultural beliefs and perceptions can be addressed and amended in families where culture is often sustained. Familial influences of dietary habits, physical activity, and obesity are discussed in the next section.

Familial Influences

Like culture, family is another aspect of the ecologic milieu in which obesity develops because familial connections are important predictors of dietary habits, physical activity, and obesity. Family preferences and roles vary among races, ethnic practices, and cultural traditions and can influence health behaviors. For example, in some Latino and Asian cultures, women serve a primary role as mother, homemaker, and caregiver. In contrast, in more westernized cultures, it is more common for both members of a spousal partnership to work outside the home. As the role of Western women in the workforce has evolved, the amount of time families eat together and at home has decreased. Now more than ever, Americans are eating out, ordering take-out meals, or bringing home fast food. Both parents often work—some long hours—and there are often few opportunities to cook healthy meals at home. These types of family roles can influence food shopping, cooking, and dining choices as well as methods and rituals (e.g., eating meals as a family), and can specifically affect children's eating habits and overall health (Bruss, Morris, & Dannison, 2003; Yuasa et al., 2008).

Some have suggested that changes in family roles, reliance on prepared or packaged food, and irregular eating patterns might contribute to weight gain, specifically among children (Strauss & Knight, 1999). Other family practices, like family dining and social rituals, can also influence health behaviors. Family rituals often develop based on particular preferences like eating certain foods on certain days of the week (e.g., pizza night) or playing sports together on particular holidays. These rituals can be both positive and negative, teaching children and other family members healthful or risky patterns and contributing to a healthy or obesogenic lifestyle as children mature (Birch & Davison, 2001). While this topic won't be explored here, it's important to keep in mind that family rituals are complicated by genetic predispositions to obesity and fat distribution (Bindon, Dressler, Gilliland, & Crews, 2007; Bouchard, 1997; Treuth, Butte, & Sorkin, 2003).

Familial Influences on Dietary Habits

Like cultural influences on dietary habits, familial influences can be important determinants of behavior. For example, dietary preferences can be influenced by familial preferences and can be influenced by parents' eating behaviors and home food environments (Birch & Davison, 2001). Parents influence children by determining their home food environments, but sometimes home food environments can reflect a reaction to children's desires and characteristics (Ventura & Birch, 2008). Even certain parenting practices have been associated with children's dietary intake and weight status. One study found that families with clear communication, proper behavior control, and structured parenting helped to regulate children's healthy behaviors (Chen & Kennedy, 2002).

Similar to cultural events, family birthdays, holidays, and other celebrations might include certain types of food that families usually prepare. Cakes, candy, and large meals are the norm for some family celebrations with second helpings sometimes encouraged. For example, if a family spends a great deal of money and time preparing a meal, they and their guests might be obligated to eat the meal and encouraged to eat additional servings.

Not only are celebration meals a familial factor for dietary habits, but the quantity of food or portion sizes can be influenced by the family (Bruss, Morris, & Dannison, 2003). If a child grows up never learning what a proper portion size is, the child may always resort to eating larger portion sizes based on what was learned from the family. Also, like celebration meals, some families encourage eating larger portions of food if a significant amount of time and money was invested in garnering and preparing the meal.

Attitudes about wasting food can be a familial influence on eating behaviors. Some families might encourage eating all the food on the plate (i.e., cleaning the plate) because of concerns about food insecurity (Olson, Bove, & Miller, 2007). For older generations, eating everything on the plate might have been seen as a necessity because of economic hardships or an overall lack of resources. Although this concept may be less apparent or emphasized today, its remnants still remain in many families and their eating habits.

The family can also influence overall food choice. Studies suggest that available food in one's home can influence the family's food choices (Birch & Davison, 2001). If more fruits and vegetables are available in the home to eat, family members might be more likely to choose these foods. Further, if a mother or father choose to eat certain types of food, children might be more likely to eat those same foods (Savage, Fisher, & Birch, 2007). How these habits transfer from childhood to adulthood is often more complex and involves other aspects of the social obesogenic environment. Although the relationships are complex and often bidirectional, healthy parent modeling, clear family communication, appropriate behavior control, and a healthy home food environment can all help children make healthier food choices.

Familial Influences on Physical Activity

Like dietary habits, the infrastructure of a family (figure 11.2) often influences physical activity types, amounts, and adherence. Depending upon the physical activity levels of members, the family can facilitate or hinder an active lifestyle.

The type of physical activity one chooses can often be linked to family preferences or traditions (Bruss et al., 2003). For many families, a holiday or

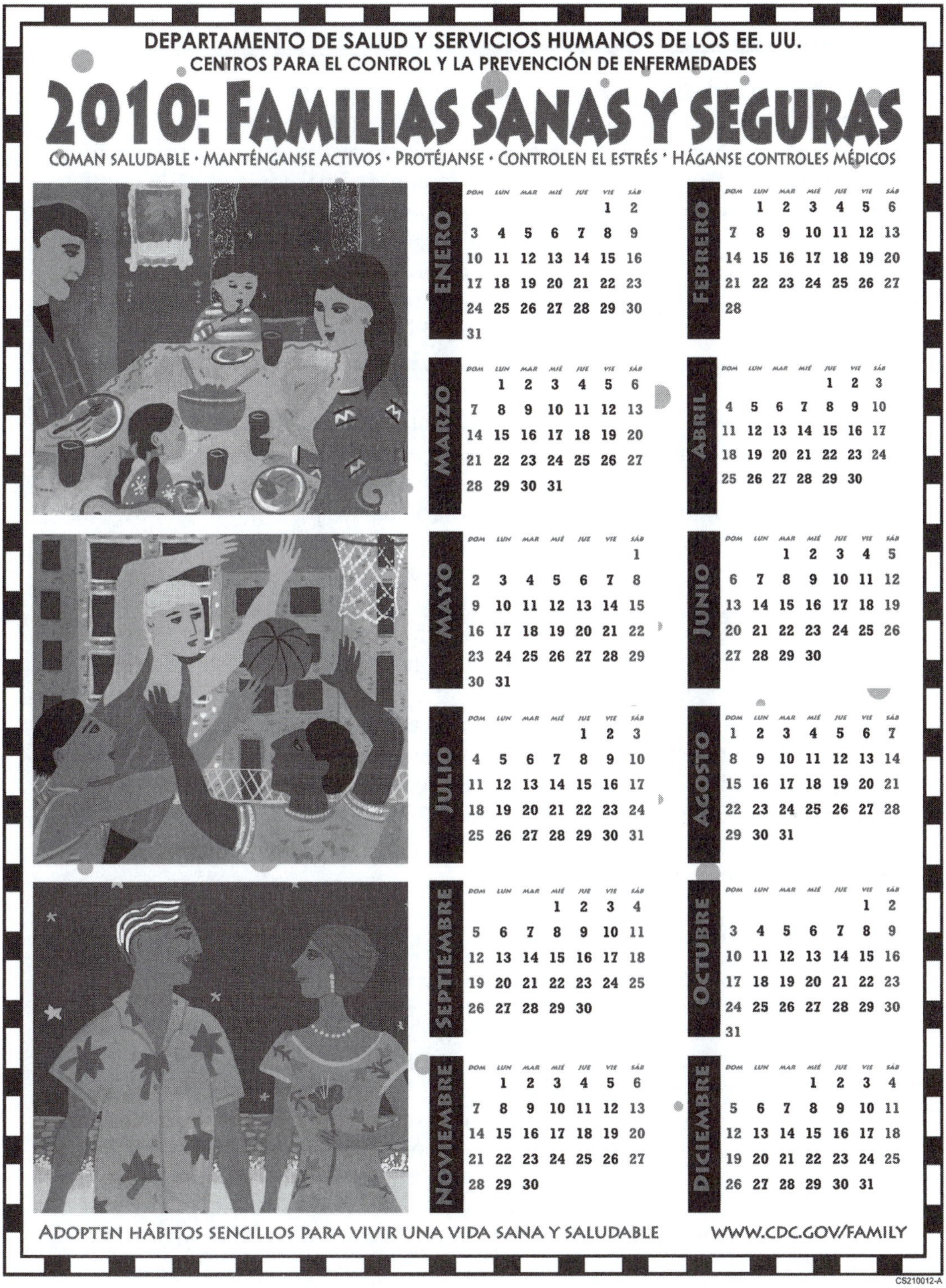

FIGURE 11.2 The CDC's *Healthy Families* campaign encourages families to eat healthfully, get regular physical activity, and spend time with family and friends. Materials are created to target people of many cultures, such as this calendar in Spanish.

U.S. Department of Health and Human Services, Centers for Disease Control and Prevention celebration can be associated with playing a certain sport. For example, playing baseball on Labor Day might be a family tradition that later influences family members' physical activity preferences. Playing baseball might be fondly remembered and associated with fun, family, and friends, so a child or other family member might be more likely to play baseball because of these types of memories. On the other hand, a child forced to play a disliked sport could resent the sport later or any physical activity associated with the sport. Like eating habits, the modes of physical activity that family members ultimately choose might have been initially modeled by other family members.

The familial social experiences and roles are also significant influences of physical activity (Khanam & Costarelli, 2008). Many families' social lives center around their children's sporting activities and the social interactions associated with them. Families might do specific physical activities because of the relationships resulting from these physical activities. For example, a father might begin to coach his daughter's soccer team to spend more time with her, which could ultimately result in more physical activity for the father. Familial roles might also allow for particular types of physical activity. A mother might join a mother-walking group, not just because of the benefits of physical activity, but because of the social interactions the mothers share. Family members sharing unique experiences with other family members might increase the likelihood of an entire family engaging in a healthy behavior and improve the intergenerational transmission of a physically active lifestyle.

Family relationships influence adherence to physical activity and other health behavior regimens. Maintaining consistent, regular physical activity in order to lose weight can be a challenging behavioral change, but some

Implementing Policy

We Can!

The National Heart, Lung, and Blood Institute (NHLBI), in collaboration with the National Institute of Diabetes and Digestive and Kidney Diseases (NIDDK), the Eunice Kennedy Shriver National Institute of Child and Human Development, and the National Cancer Institute (NCI), have collaborated to create *We Can!* (Ways to Enhance Children's Activity and Nutrition). This national movement is designed to give parents, caregivers, and communities tools to help children ages 8 to 13 to stay at a healthy weight. *We Can!* provides parents and caregivers with fun activities that encourage healthy eating, more physical activity, and less time sitting in front of television or computer screens. *We Can!* also offers organizations, community groups, and health professionals a centralized resource to promote a healthy weight in youth through community outreach, partnership development, and media activities that can be adapted to meet the needs of diverse populations. Science-based educational programs, support materials, training opportunities, and other resources are available to support programming for youth, parents, and families in the community (USDHHS, 2010).

family-based treatment methods have shown success in overweight white children (Epstein, Valoski, Koeske, & Wing, 1986). Family members often provide support by providing transportation to a physical activity resource, watching a family member engage in physical activity, or joining the family member in the activity. These supportive behaviors vary, but adherence to a physical activity is more likely to occur if there is social support for the behavior change (Richter et al., 2002; Wilbur et al., 2003).

Interactions Between Family and Culture

Familial and cultural influences on dietary habits, physical activity, and obesity are often interrelated. Although the family itself is a predictor of dietary habits and physical activity, family practices can differ depending upon the culture of a family. Also, culture can interact with familial influences on health behaviors, often as a guiding force for family behaviors. For example, data suggest that a black mother's viewpoint of her daughter's body can have a positive influence on the daughter's body image satisfaction (Thomas & James, 1988), which could have positive benefits for health behaviors for black females (Melnyk & Weinstein, 1994). Similarly, if a Latina mother eats particular foods common in her culture, she might cook these same foods for her family, regardless of the family's primary cultural affiliation or practices. In these two examples, culture and family are interrelated, and both can influence health behaviors that can prevent or reverse obesity.

❑ Distinguish among culture, race, and ethnicity.
❑ Describe cultural factors that might influence obesity.
❑ Describe familial factors that might influence obesity.

GETTING STARTED

Summary

As scientists and clinicians attempt to investigate and treat the obesity epidemic, cultural and familial influences on physical activity, dietary habits, and obesity have emerged as complex yet significant influences on dietary habits, physical activity, and obesity. Obesity can also vary by ethnicity. Culture can affect health beliefs and body perceptions, which can, in turn, cause obesity. Family roles and relationships influence members' dietary habits and physical activity choices, especially those of children. Some family-based obesity treatment methods have had success in some populations, and national organizations have joined forces to educate families and caregivers on health behaviors. Finally, family and culture are often interrelated and should be considered individually and collectively when examining and repairing social aspects of obesogenic environments.

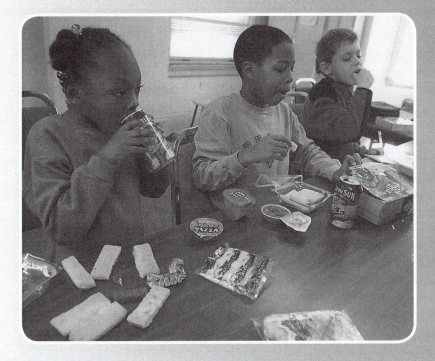

CHAPTER 12

Social Justice, Health Disparities, and Obesity

As the obesity epidemic steadily increases in the United States, of particular concern are populations of color and those with low socioeconomic status (SES) or social class who are most vulnerable to obesity and related health-compromising conditions (Ogden et al., 2006). Some scholars suggest that there may be systematic differences in environmental factors and social inequalities that contribute to these disparities (Braveman & Gruskin, 2003). Further evidence suggests that the health and life expectancy of American racial and ethnic minorities is lower than the general population even when controlling for income (Prus, 2007). Social injustices can include decreased access to health care, physical activity resources, healthful food options, high quality education opportunities, safe and quality housing, and occupational opportunities (*Access to Healthy Foods in Low-Income Neighborhoods, Opportunities for Public Policy,* 2008; Braveman et al., 2005; Lee & Cubbin, 2009) and can also be dependent on geographical location, like rural settings (Lee et al., 2007). Systematic disadvantages at both individual and environmental levels are recurring in health disparities (Lee & Cubbin, 2009).

Social justice in health is defined as equality or similarity in health and its determinants, regardless of one's position in a social hierarchy (Braveman & Gruskin, 2003). A corollary of social justice is that good health is a right, rather than a privilege, for everyone; everyone, regardless of social advantage, has the same opportunities to be healthy (Link & Phelan, 2002). The history of a society contributes to social justice, meaning that past social justices or injustices, like discrimination or oppression, contribute to current disparities. As a result of the complexity and historical underpinnings, current social injustices are often very difficult to describe, quantify, and remedy.

Despite these challenges, data suggest in general that populations of color, those with lower SES, and women tend to have higher rates of obesity and lower rates of physical activity. Some social injustices that scholars have suggested are higher stress; less leisure time; and less access to goods, services, and other resources that support physical activity, healthful dietary habits, and healthy body weights (Lee & Cubbin, 2009). Taken together, these factors provide significant barriers to physical activity and result in systematic disparities in physical activity and its related health outcomes (figure 12.1). This chapter discusses, in association with the obesogenic environment, issues such as inequalities in access to health care, education, occupational opportunities, and quality housing in safe neighborhoods. Social justice plays an important role in health and in the ability to maintain a healthy body weight conceptualized at both individual and environmental levels.

The development of health disparities is typically a slow process that may occur over centuries. As a clear example, in the United States the history of racial discrimination and oppression has contributed to current social inequalities in health among African Americans. The history of oppression has contributed to overrepresentation of blacks in lower SES, residential segregation, and chronic stress (Williams & Collins, 1995). These effects can

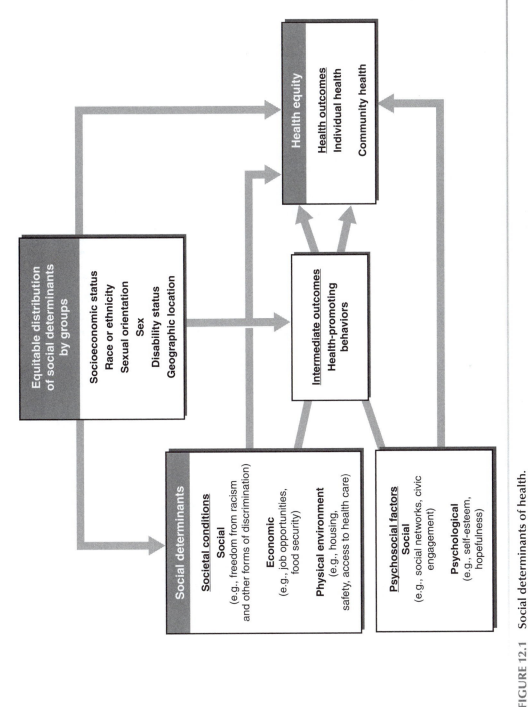

FIGURE 12.1 Social determinants of health.

Reprinted from L.K. Brennan Ramirez, E.A. Baker, and M. Metzler, 2008, *Promoting health equity: A resource to help communities address social determinants of health* (Atlanta: Centers for Disease Control and Prevention), 10. Figure adapted from Blue Cross and Blue Shield of Minnesota Foundation, n.d., and Anderson et al., 2003.

be seen clearly even today, in the twenty-first century. Compared to whites, blacks are more likely to have received an inferior high school education, are paid less for a given level of education, accumulate less wealth over the lifespan, and are more likely to experience unemployment (Braveman et al., 2005). Throughout this chapter, discussion of the correlates of health should be considered in the context of the reality that some groups are overburdened by disparities through no immediate fault of their own or others, but rather through the consequences of a history of oppression, misinformation, and misunderstanding.

Socioeconomic Status

Socioeconomic status (SES) refers to relative social position and can be measured at the individual level and neighborhood level. Education level, occupation, income, wealth, and place of residence all contribute to one's SES. Although not all of these factors may influence individual SES, one or several usually influence social position or social class. Each of the determinants of SES are discussed below.

Education is a major determinant of future employment opportunities because individuals with higher education levels typically have higher employment income (U.S. Department of Education National Center for Education Statistics, 2008). Area of residence often determines which school a child will attend, and thus it may be considered a primary sequential determinant of SES. Although not always the case, lower SES neighborhoods often have lower quality school districts (Muijs, Harris, Chapman, Stoll, & Russ, 2004). Since the residents of lower SES neighborhoods often have fewer individual resources themselves, they may not be able to afford private or special schooling for children. It is often the case that children are groomed as early as middle school for college. Schools that offer inferior quality education, in turn, provide fewer opportunities for a college education.

Education often determines one's occupation, which in turn determines income. Because income can contribute to the amount of education one can afford, and education, in turn, contributes to the amount of income one can make, SES is often complex and cyclical.

SES, Social Injustices, Health Behaviors, and Obesity

Physical inactivity and obesity continue to be more prevalent among those with lower individual socioeconomic status (SES) and those who live in lower SES neighborhoods (USDHHS, 1996) indicating significant health disparities. In contrast, in other countries where there has been more recent industrialization, obesity is actually associated with higher SES (Popkin & Doak, 1998; Wang, 2001). The nature of the relationship between SES and obesity is not always clearly understood. Factors of SES influence health directly (through education, income, place of residence, and so on) and indirectly. For example, social position affects exposure to life events, chronic stressors, and health-related lifestyle preferences (Prus, 2007). Furthermore, individuals with limited material and psychosocial resources tend to have more chronic disease and shorter life spans (Adler et al., 1994). Health disadvantages attached to early risky and lower SES lifestyles also cumulate with age. The higher one's SES, the longer the life span, and health inequalities between SES groups follow a similar pattern of divergence. The relationships among the determinants of individual SES, neighborhood SES, social injustices, and health behaviors that can prevent or cause obesity are discussed below.

Educational Attainment

In the United States, along with most industrialized nations, educational attainment is consistently associated with health behaviors and health outcomes. It is unclear which leads to improved health outcomes: the sheer increase in knowledge that comes with greater education, or the greater income that is associated with increased education. Lower educational attainment may contribute to lower health literacy. According to Healthy People 2010, health literacy is "the degree to which individuals have the capacity to obtain, process, and understand basic health information and services needed to make appropriate health decisions" (National Network of Libraries of Medicine, 2010). Health literacy is important for understanding how health behaviors like nutrition and physical activity are prioritized (Health Resources and Services Administration, 2008). Since

> Health Literacy = the ability to obtain, process, and understand basic health information needed to make decisions and follow instructions for treatment.

nutrition and physical activity recommendations periodically change, frequent education is necessary for the most up-to-date information. Obese patients with low levels of literacy are less likely to understand the adverse health consequences of obesity and the need to lose excess body weight (Kennen et al., 2005). In addition, low health literacy also likely contributes to misunderstanding about why health recommendations change. Many people do not understand that scientific discovery is dynamic and colored by political priorities, and recommendations that reflected the state of the science or what was politically palatable five or ten years ago are no longer up to date.

Another compounding factor associated with lower educational attainment is that people with lower educational attainment may be more likely to work more hours a week, further hindering opportunities for increasing healthy behaviors like physical activity, proper sleep, and healthier home-cooked meals. Education is a major determinant of future employment opportunities since individuals with higher education typically are employed in higher income positions (U.S. Department of Education National Center for Education Statistics, 2008).

Occupational Status

Like education, occupation is also a major determinant of SES and health. A person's occupation can influence the amount of recreation time and resources available and potential levels of stress (Martinez & Fischer, 2009). In addition, because people in positions of lower SES are sometimes prone to longer work days (Artazcoz, Cortes, Escriba-Aguir, Cascant, & Villegas, 2009), there is less time for rest and recreation, further contributing to stress. Not only do these longer work hours leave less time to relax, but there is also less time for practicing other healthy behaviors like getting adequate sleep, spending time with family and friends, and preparing and eating healthful meals.

Those in positions of lower SES may have fewer work options and may face longer commute times because affordable housing may not be close to the worksite. Longer commutes by personal vehicle have been associated with higher rates of obesity (Frank, Andresen, & Schmid, 2004). Longer commutes by public transportation may add physical activity to one's life, potentially reducing obesity, but the trade-off in time away from the home can counter the potential protective benefit of active transportation (Bassett et al., 2008; Lee & Cubbin, 2009; McDonald, 2007; Rosenberg, Sallis, Conway, Cain, & McKenzie, 2006).

Work environments may not promote healthful behaviors. Many jobs require sitting at a desk with reliance on computer and phone rather than physical activity. In the service industry, where many people of lower SES work (Boushey, Fremstad, Gragg, & Waller, 2007; Dodson & Bravo, 2005), there may be physical activity involved such as serving food, assisting customers in a store, or providing some other service; however, the mental and physical demand of these positions make for very high stress levels that may reduce the protective effect of any physical activity done while on the job (Ehrenreich, 2001). Furthermore, due to the low wages offered in these positions, many people find it necessary to hold more than one job. The resulting longer hours and convenience of fast food can contribute to unhealthy habits leading to overweight and obesity.

Income and Wealth

Income and wealth are often major contributors to good health and obesity prevention. Income is the payment of money in exchange for goods or services rendered, while wealth refers to the accumulation of valuable possessions, resources, and property. Wealth is important because it determines security and insures consistency of lifestyle in times of both societal plenty and poverty. Income and wealth improve health by improving nutritional quality and reducing stress. As income increases, there are also increases in leisure time, and access to physical activity resources, healthcare, and nutritious foods can also increase (Lee & Cubbin, 2009).

Those with higher income and greater wealth have better standards of living compared to those with lower incomes and less wealth. They command more opportunities to improve and maintain health, such as access to wellness facilities or centers, advanced medical resources, and quality healthcare facilities. They tend to have permanent homes, excellent sanitation facilities, and assistance in completing excess or unwanted tasks such as supplemental child care, housekeeping, financial accounting, groundskeeping, shopping, and other tasks. The higher standard of living allows for more leisure time as well as access to resources and behaviors that support healthful dietary habits such as the time and resources to prepare and eat healthful foods, get sufficient recreational physical activity, and maintain preventive health care. All these, singly and in combination, contribute to reducing obesity and its detrimental effects.

A higher income improves nutrition. It allows for the purchase of higher quality, nutritionally dense, freshly produced food that may cost more than cheaply produced food with high energy density and low nutritional value. Compared to packaged and canned foods, fresh produce is usually more expensive (Morland & Filomena, 2007). Higher-quality produce, such as organically grown or "hot house" produce, is even more expensive, further hindering healthful eating for lower income individuals and families. Prepackaged and canned foods allow for longer shelf life but also have additional ingredients like partially hydrogenized oils and high fructose corn syrup, both of which can have negative health implications (e.g., increased blood cholesterol and blood sugar) (Loera, 2009). Those with more wealth have more options concerning these prepackaged foods: they may choose to store them, eat them if desired, or distribute them to those who may need them.

All of these factors help to reduce stress both on a daily basis and over the life span. Those with more wealth need not worry about whether there will be sufficient food for dinner or figure out how to buy the most amount of food for the lowest price. There is no concern with whether there will be enough work to generate income necessary to pay the rent or repair appliances should they break. Over the course of a life span, those with higher incomes typically have more opportunities for recreation and rest, which decreases stress levels. Stress has been associated with obesity, and those who can reduce it tend to live longer, healthier lives (Henry, 1988).

Neighborhood SES

Although people tend to live near friends and relatives, in many cases, there may be little choice involved in neighborhood of residence. In many places in the world, neighborhood of residence is regulated either directly by the government or indirectly by policies or attitudes favoring residential segregation. For example, in the United States, neighborhoods are still often segregated by race or ethnicity, partly because of a long history of housing discrimination. In the United States, migrant populations and populations of color, such as African Americans and Latinos, as well as female-headed households, are more likely to live in lower SES neighborhoods compared to whites (Cubbin, Hadden, & Winkleby, 2001).

In the United States and other countries, migrant and ethnic minority populations are often overrepresented among those of lower SES. A minority population is defined as a racial or ethnic group thought to be different from the larger group of which it is part. Minority populations in the United States include African American, Latino, Asian, American Indian, Alaska Native, Native Hawaiian, and other Pacific Islander groups. It is now the case that Latino populations have increased in size to become the dominant population in some areas of the Unites States (U.S. Census Bureau, 2009).

Neighborhood of residence has been associated with health behaviors and outcomes, including obesity and related behaviors (Cubbin et al., 2001; Cubbin et al., 2006; Lee & Cubbin, 2002). Although the mechanisms are not well understood, study after study has demonstrated an association between neighborhood and health, regardless of individual SES. Neighborhoods influence the health behaviors and outcomes of all residents, regardless of individual characteristics, because all individuals share the same neighborhood social and physical features. Residence in a lower SES neighborhood may mean reduced access to goods and services and greater daily stress, both contributing to obesity.

Lower SES neighborhoods are characterized as deprived of capital and resources because of a myriad of contributing factors. These include fewer individually owned homes, more transient residents, a lower tax base for municipal improvements, and less social and political power to demand improvements. Many lower SES neighborhoods have substandard housing, safety concerns, and fewer healthcare opportunities (Lee & Cubbin, 2009).

Higher SES neighborhoods are often safer and cleaner with more physical activity and healthful eating opportunities. Higher SES neighborhoods may have better schools that, in turn, contribute to improved education. Healthcare resources, such as doctors' offices and hospitals, are also more likely to be located in higher SES areas. An increasing number of quality hospitals and specialized practices are leaving low SES cities and towns and relocating to suburban areas (Nandi & Harris, 1999).

Higher SES neighborhoods may have more physical activity opportunities. Several studies suggest that physical activity resources are better quality and more accessible in higher SES neighborhoods (Estabrooks, Lee, & Gyurcsik, 2003; Heinrich et al., 2008; Lee, Booth, Reese-Smith, Regan, & Howard, 2005).

What are some things neighborhood residents can do to empower themselves and their neighborhood, and what are some actions residents can take to create healthier environments in their neighborhood?

Accessible physical activity resources are those resources that are free for use (e.g., most public parks, trails, basketball courts, etc.). Inaccessible physical activity resources could include gyms that require membership fees, skating rinks that charge admission, and sports clubs that require annual dues (Lee et al., 2005). Quality, in terms of poor aesthetic appeal and many incivilities in physical activity resources, is a predictor of both obesity prevalence and physical activity in low-income minority populations, suggesting that accessibility may be an advantage in higher SES neighborhoods with greater aesthetic appeal and fewer incivilities (Heinrich et al., 2008). Having accessible physical activity resources to use is an important determinant of health behaviors.

Weight Discrimination

Weight discrimination may be one of the last acceptable forms of intolerance in our society (Puhl & Brownell, 2003). Obese and overweight persons may be more vulnerable to discrimination in a variety of domains compared to their underweight counterparts, and their personal coping mechanisms are typically understudied (Puhl & Brownell, 2003). Weight discrimination can affect overweight and obese people socially and professionally and can even determine the quality of health care received.

Overweight and obese persons are discriminated against in many social environments. Studies have shown that obese persons report being stared at and verbally harassed while walking down the street, exercising in public, and eating out at restaurants (Cossrow, Jeffery, & McGuire, 2001). Other negative social situations caused by weight discrimination include friendship and dating. In one study, an obese woman reported, "But they don't realize that it's kind of hard when you already are [overweight], to get someone to love you that way . . . I'm a lot nicer than a lot of other people in the world that have boyfriends and girlfriends" (Cossrow et al., 2001, p. 211). Many studies have shown that weight discrimination in employment settings is a common issue for the overweight and obese. Obese individuals report higher employment discrimination, which may lead to adverse physical and psychological outcomes (Roehling, Roehling, & Pichler, 2007). Employment discrimination can affect work decisions, performance, and attitudes.

The obese are also more likely to report unfair treatment from health care providers specifically due to their body weight (Cossrow et al., 2001). One study found that some doctors only addressed an obese individual's weight problem, despite other existing conditions (Cossrow et al., 2001). Other studies have found that up to 50% of doctors have negative stereotypes of obese individuals (Foster et al., 2003) and some obese patients are offered shorter-than-average consultations by physicians (Hebl & Xu, 2001).

The prevalence of weight discrimination is increasing in the United States. Although other forms of discrimination have decreased over recent years, weight discrimination has increased by 66% from 1995 to 2006 (Andreyeva, Puhl, & Brownell, 2008). Weight discrimination surpasses other individual factors like ethnicity, age, education, and occupation. These data and the implication of social injustices based on weight status suggest a dire need for more pragmatic study and systematic reform.

Resiliency to Social Injustices

Many cultures have demonstrated great resiliency in the face of social injustices and systematic adverse health outcomes. Current social theories suggest that certain aspects of cultures may enhance resiliency in the face of adverse circumstances. For example, one study found that, compared to whites, African Americans were more mentally resilient in the face of greater social inequality and exposure to discrimination as well as to high rates of physical morbidity (Keyes, 2009). Factors like social resources, family relationships, and religiosity may enhance resilience in Latino cultures (Marin & Marin, 1991). In contrast, psychosocial and resiliency factors may also contribute to health disparities associated with broad sociocultural factors like low SES or minority ethnicity (Gallo, Penedo, Espinosa de los Monteros, & Arguelles, 2009).

> What are the potential unexpected consequences of efforts to reduce health disparities?

Solutions

Social injustices must be addressed in order to repair current health disparities and tackle America's obesity epidemic. The presence of systematic health disparities between social groups is evident and contributes to an obesogenic environment. Many community leaders and policy makers have begun taking action against national health disparities (figure 12.2). States like California have used policies to build parks and develop programs in lower SES neighborhoods. Other government organizations, like the Center for Disease Control and Prevention (CDC), are also working with local communities to build and repair parks in low SES neighborhoods (CDC, 2009). Many policies and urban planning methods have become effective means of preventing and treating systematic social injustices.

Social justice research has emerged as a hot topic among health and obesity research. Because of significant national health disparities, researchers are beginning to systematically document and explore determinants and consequences of social inequalities. Research institutions like the National Institutes of Health and the Centers for Population Health and Health Disparities are affiliated with various universities nationally and often focus on underserved populations like minorities and women while incorporating various disciplines and conceptual frameworks (NIH Centers for Population Health and Health Disparities, 2009). Health research and promotion addressing social justice and health disparities have become important tools when creating and enforcing public policies. It is also important to ensure that research findings are disseminated to as wide of an audience as possible. However, there is no easy solution for the problem of social injustice. Coordinated and consistent efforts must be made across a range of settings and include political, corporate, and citizen leadership and support.

PROMISING STRATEGIES

HIV/AIDS:
Improve recognition of risk, detection of infection, and referral to follow-up care; assure proper treatment; and counsel about avoiding risky behaviors.

Diabetes:
Reduce the rate of diabetes and its complications among high-risk populations, increase early detection and treatment, and increase efforts on diabetes self-management through outreach and education.

Asthma:
Reduce the frequency and severity of asthma attacks through appropriate medical care, monitoring of symptoms and objective measures of lung function, along with environmental control measures to reduce exposures to allergens and other asthma triggers.

Adult Immunization:
Promote effective provider-based intervention, increase community demand, enhance access to services, and encourage vaccination-related efforts in non-medical settings.

WHAT YOU CAN DO

Healthcare Providers
Advise and encourage clients to reduce their risk for chronic and infectious illnesses.

Ensure that standing orders are in place for screening tests.

Advise seniors and medically compromised clients to get pneumococcal and influenza vaccinations.

Conduct foot and kidney exams with diabetic clients during routine healthcare visits and recommend eye screenings annually.

Provide culturally competent and linguistically appropriate care.

Individuals
Think prevention -- see a healthcare provider annually, even if you feel healthy.

Eat more fruits and vegetables and less fat and sugar.

Get at least 30 minutes of physical activity daily -- taking the stairs burns 5 times more calories than taking the elevator.

Take loved ones to a healthcare provider.

Stop smoking.

Community
Join with others to promote community-wide health activities and campaigns.

Form coalitions with civic, professional, religious, and educational organizations to advocate health policies, programs, and services.

Support policies that promote health-care access for all.

MORE INFORMATION

CDC's Office of Minority Health and Health Disparities (OMHD)
http://www.cdc.gov/omhd/Populations/HL/hl.htm
(404) 498-2320

CDC en Español
http://www.cdc.gov/spanish/
Public Inquiry Main Line: (800) 311-3435

HHS' Office of Minority Health Resource Center (HHS OMHRC)
http://www.omhrc.gov/OMHRC/index.htm
(800) 444-6472

National Center on Minority Health and Health Disparities (NCMHD)
http://ncmhd.nih.gov
(301) 402-1366   TTY: (301) 451-9532

Firstgov en Español
http://www.firstgov.gov/Espanol/index.shtml
(800) FED-INFO (333-4636)

Seguro Social en Español
http://www.ssa.gov/espanol/
(800) 772-1213   TTY: (800) 325-0778

National Hispanic Medical Association (NHMA)
http://home.earthlink.net/~nhma/
(202) 628-5895

National Association of Hispanic Nurses (NAHN)
http://www.thehispanicnurses.org/
(202) 387-2477

FIGURE 12.2   There are many steps that can be taken to help alleviate disparities in health care among social groups. This page of a brochure from the CDC gives some tips on how people from different sectors can address the issues.

U.S. Department of Health and Human Services, Centers for Disease Control and Prevention, Office of Minority Health and Health Disparities

Implementing Policy

Community Foundations

A community foundation is a tax-exempt public charity created by and for the people in a local area. Grants are then made from these funds to nonprofit groups in order to meet the charitable goals of the donor (Marin Community Foundation, 2009). One organization in California, the Marin Community Foundation, provides community grants for access to parks and open spaces and supports projects that increase the access that low-income and minority individuals have to parks (Marin Community Foundation, 2009). While open space and agricultural lands are at risk from the pressures of sprawl, the Marin Community Foundation aims to protect these areas by providing ongoing stewardship and restoration. In particular, this organization also helps underserved residents use and benefit from natural areas, parks, and other green spaces throughout Marin County. Underserved residents include people with low incomes, people of color, youth, persons with mobility impairment, and older adults. Marin Community Foundation funds grants that develop, refine, and implement green space programming that is culturally relevant and meets the needs of underserved residents. It also supports community-based planning for existing and new green spaces to benefit underserved communities (Marin Community Foundation, 2009).

GETTING STARTED

❏ Recognize socioeconomic disadvantages affecting certain groups in the population and describe how these originate and persist.
❏ Describe neighborhood and individual socioeconomic status (SES).
❏ Explain the relationships between SES, the obesogenic environment, and individual health.
❏ Recognize systematic oppression in neighborhood and individual health.

Summary

Minority and low SES populations are most vulnerable to obesity and related health-compromising conditions. SES refers to relative social position; it is determined by education level, occupation, income, place of residence, and wealth. SES can be measured at the individual level and neighborhood level. Systematic disparities in environmental factors and social inequalities can contribute to social injustices like decreased access to health care, physical activity resources, healthful food options, high quality education opportunities, safe and quality housing, and occupational opportunities. Social injustices based on weight status are also increasing, suggesting a need for more pragmatic study and systematic reform. Health research and promotion addressing social justice and health disparities have become an important tool when creating and enforcing public policies, but there is no easy solution. Coordinated and consistent efforts must be made in a variety of domains in order to prevent and treat social injustices, such as health disparities, that can lead to obesity.

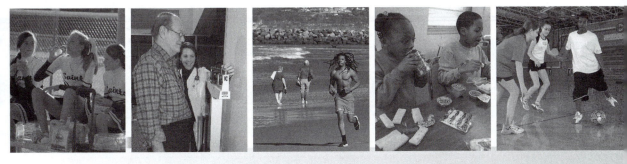

Media and Marketing

The last part of this book is by no means the least important! Media and marketing are pervasive elements in our daily lives. Most of us can remember a musical jingle advertising a favorite cereal or other food from childhood, demonstrating the staying power of a strong advertising campaign. Media and marketing are increasingly using advanced technology, and so we include some information on technology in this part of the book as well. Many examples in this part have to do with food and the food industry, but physical activity is also relevant here. The U.S. National Physical Activity Plan (2010) offers recommendations and suggestions specifically targeting the media as an important factor influencing physical activity . We devote an entire part of the book to media and marketing because they are very important determinants of dietary habits and physical activity. Readers will see examples in this part that will connect them back to the previous chapters that look at food technology, the emergence of the obesogenic environment, and policy, among others. Media and marketing are here to stay, and it's time to take a long look at their potential role in reversing the obesogenic environment.

PART

five

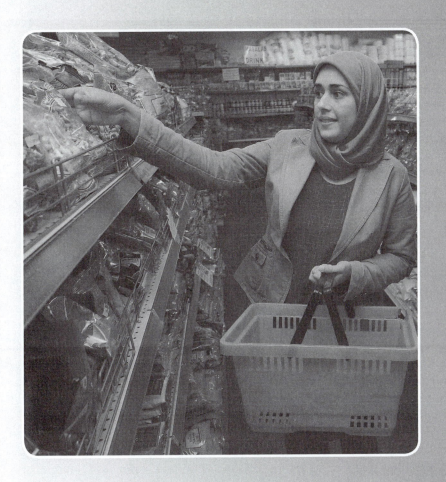

CHAPTER 13

Point of Purchase

The retail point of purchase is the place where goods or services are purchased by the consumer (American Marketing Association, 2009). In the case of food, the retail point of purchase is typically a store or restaurant, but it may include any place where food is sold or served. This chapter focuses on food, dietary habits, consumers, and how they are linked to food marketing at the retail point of purchase.

In most cases, consumers have a general idea of what they intend to purchase when they go to a store or restaurant. They may have a list of items that they use weekly, which may include staple items needing replacement and special occasion items for a special recipe or event (figure 13.1). At the restaurant, people often have a few favorites that they typically order. Marketing materials, such as advertisements or special promotions, are designed with this information in mind. Most people, about 70% according to marketing surveys, have not decided on a particular brand when they walk in the supermarket door (Meyers Research Center, 1995). So, if a consumer is going to buy a jar of peanut butter, when he gets to the store, he first looks for the peanut butter aisle or section and then chooses among the available brands and styles based on a variety of factors. Deciding which brand and style to purchase may not occur until he arrives at the store and investigates the options. Exceptions may be made for brand loyalty or possession of coupons for specific products. However, even in these exceptions, many consumers may change their decision based on new information gleaned at the point of purchase.

Point of purchase = the location where commodities are sold by the retailer to the consumer.

Marketing, Advertising, Branding

The information that may be relevant at the point of purchase may include marketing materials, advertising, and branding information, along with simple product information provided on the label. Marketing encompasses the entire process of recruiting and retaining customers (American Marketing Association, 2009). Advertising is communication from the company to the consumer about the product, and branding refers to the process of associating a name, icon, or other piece of information with a particular product (American Marketing Association, 2009).

Marketing is a cornerstone of consumerism; it is used to increase product availability and visibility and to increase brand awareness. For example, marketing may be used by an industry group to increase product availability and visibility, and a company may focus more on increasing awareness of its particular brand. The fundamental goal of marketing is to stimu-

How do people decide which products to purchase at a store or restaurant?

My Shopping List

Make a shopping list. Include the items you need for your menus and any low-calorie basics you need to restock in your kitchen.

Dairy Case

- ☐ Fat-free (skim) or low-fat (1%) milk
- ☐ Low-fat or reduced fat cottage cheese
- ☐ Fat-free cottage cheese
- ☐ Low-fat or reduced fat cheeses
- ☐ Fat-free or low-fat yogurt
- ☐ Light or diet margarine (tub, squeeze, or spray)
- ☐ Fat-free or reduced fat sour cream
- ☐ Fat-free cream cheese
- ☐ Eggs/egg substitute
- ☐ _____

Breads, Muffins, and Rolls

- ☐ Bread, bagels, or pita bread
- ☐ English muffins
- ☐ Yeast breads (whole wheat, rye, pumpernickel, multi-grain, or raisin)
- ☐ Corn tortillas (not fried)
- ☐ Low-fat flour tortillas
- ☐ Fat-free biscuit mix
- ☐ Rice crackers
- ☐ Challah
- ☐ _____

Cereals, Crackers, Rice, Noodles, and Pasta

- ☐ Plain cereal, dry or cooked
- ☐ Saltines, soda crackers (low-sodium or unsalted tops)
- ☐ Graham crackers
- ☐ Other low-fat crackers
- ☐ Rice (brown, white, etc.)
- ☐ Pasta (noodles, spaghetti)
- ☐ Bulgur, couscous, or kasha
- ☐ Potato mixes (made without fat)
- ☐ Wheat mixes
- ☐ Tabouli grain salad

- ☐ Hominy
- ☐ Polenta
- ☐ Polvillo
- ☐ Hominy grits
- ☐ Quinoa
- ☐ Millet
- ☐ Aramanth
- ☐ Oatmeal
- ☐ _____

Meat Case

- ☐ White meat chicken and turkey (skin off)
- ☐ Fish (not battered)
- ☐ Beef, round or sirloin
- ☐ Extra lean ground beef such as ground round
- ☐ Pork tenderloin
- ☐ 95% fat-free lunch meats or low-fat deli meats
- ☐ _____

Meat Equivalents:

- ☐ Tofu (or bean curd)
- ☐ Beans (see bean list)
- ☐ Eggs/egg substitutes (see dairy list)
- ☐ _____

Fruit (fresh, canned, and frozen)

Fresh Fruit:

- ☐ Apples
- ☐ Bananas
- ☐ Peaches
- ☐ Oranges
- ☐ Pears
- ☐ Grapes
- ☐ Grapefruit
- ☐ Apricots
- ☐ Dried Fruits
- ☐ Cherries
- ☐ Plums

- ☐ Melons
- ☐ Lemons
- ☐ Limes
- ☐ Plantains
- ☐ Mangoes
- ☐ _____

Exotic Fresh Fruit:

- ☐ Kiwi
- ☐ Olives
- ☐ Figs
- ☐ Quinces
- ☐ Currants
- ☐ Persimmons
- ☐ Pomegranates
- ☐ Papaya
- ☐ Zapote
- ☐ Guava
- ☐ Starfruit
- ☐ Litchi nuts
- ☐ Winter melons
- ☐ _____

Canned Fruit (in juice or water):

- ☐ Canned pineapple
- ☐ Applesauce
- ☐ Other canned fruits (mixed or plain)
- ☐ _____

Frozen Fruits (without added sugar):

- ☐ Blueberries
- ☐ Raspberries
- ☐ 100% fruit juice
- ☐ _____

Dried Fruit:

- ☐ Raisins/dried fruit (these tend to be higher in calories than fresh fruit)
- ☐ _____

FIGURE 13.1 Using a shopping list, such as this one from A Healthier You, can help keep consumers from making impulsive purchases and falling victim to marketing and advertising. For the full shopping list, go to www.health.gov/dietaryguidelines/dga2005/healthieryou/pdf/shopping_list.pdf.

Reprinted from U.S. Department of Health and Human Services, Office of Disease Prevention and Health Promotion, 2005, *A healthier you: Based on the Dietary Guidelines for Americans* (Washington, DC: U.S. Department of Health and Human Services), 107-108.

late product trial and purchase. Marketing is used to help customers make informed buying decisions, and at the point of purchase, to encourage impulse buys—unplanned or spontaneous purchases—typically for items not on the list. Marketing can be a powerful force on consumers by creating a unified brand image in multiple locations and has been shown to increase sales. For example, in our peanut butter example, the consumer may see a particular brand of peanut butter advertised on the television and later find a coupon for the same brand in the newspaper. During the weekly grocery shopping trip, perhaps that same brand is having a special promotion at the store. In this example, the coordinated marketing has increased product awareness and visibility as well as awareness of the particular brand. This awareness may then stimulate the consumer to buy the brand, possibly generating brand loyalty if the consumer is satisfied with the product.

Although multinational corporations have used marketing to great success in the arena of snack foods, there have been relatively few strategies tested to market more nutritionally dense foods like fruits and vegetables. In particular, fresh fruits and vegetables, unless they are supported by a particular advocacy group—for example, the Florida Avocado Administrative Committee—may have little coordinated marketing. Coordinated efforts at marketing healthful foods by linking standard guidelines for healthy eating to the particular food that satisfies guidelines would likely increase consumption of these foods.

Advertising is a one-way, or unidirectional, form of communication from a company to consumers, paid for by the company itself. Advertising is done in an effort to persuade consumers to buy a particular product, brand, or service. It is delivered through many communication channels, including media, signs, and product placement (figure 13.2). At the retail point of purchase, advertising can include signs, but it may also include other promotional materials like point-of-purchase discounts, free samples, product placement, or other strategies. For instance, companies pay slotting fees to insure that

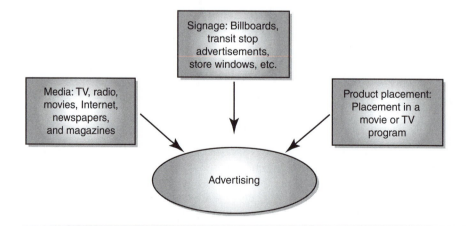

FIGURE 13.2 Communication channels of advertising.

their products are placed at eye level for potential consumers ("Who's Minding the Shelves?," 2000).

A brand is a name, icon, or other piece of information that is associated with a particular product or service (American Marketing Association, 2009). A good brand is easy to understand and recognize: It simply describes the product or service in an engaging format. Brands are very important for increasing recognition of that product or service; their goal is to increase consumer loyalty. Consumer loyalty is important for reliable sales; thus, branding is very important in marketing. There are companies and services devoted entirely to brand development: These services create, test, and implement brands. A good brand may not only increase consumer loyalty but may also serve other marketing needs, like stimulating trial of the product.

The Four Ps

The four Ps of retail point-of-purchase marketing are product, pricing, promotion, and placement (figure 13.3). Product refers to the specifications of the good or services itself. These are typically described on the label of the product. Pricing is the product cost that the consumer actually pays. Promotion refers to any publicity, advertising, or selling strategies that are associated with the product. Placement refers to how the product is made available for the consumer.

Product specifications are provided on the product label and can include a list of ingredients; nutrition information, which is required in the United States by the Food and Drug Administration; and branding, marketing, or advertising information. Ingredient lists start with the product ingredient that is present in the highest amount in the product, and follow sequentially to the last item present in the lowest amount in the product (USDHHS, 2009). For example, in our peanut butter example, the list of ingredients might read "Peanuts, dextrose, hydrogenated vegetable oil (cotton seed and/or rapeseed), salt." This means that in this product, the most plentiful ingredient is peanuts, and the

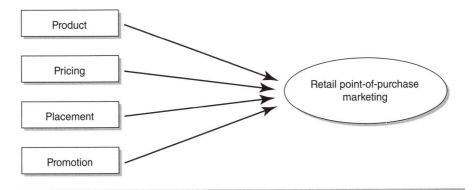

FIGURE 13.3 Four Ps of retail point-of-purchase marketing.

Implementing Policy

Advertising Food to Children

As research continues to demonstrate the negative effects food marketing has on childhood obesity, the Federal Trade Commission (FTC), the Food and Drug Administration (FDA), the United States Department of Agriculture (USDA), and the Centers for Disease Control and Prevention (CDC) have collaborated to issue a set of proposed standards for food marketing to children. Proposed food advertising recommendations include marketing only 100% fruits and vegetables or fruit and vegetable juice in all forms; marketing foods that make a meaningful contribution to a child's diet; and marketing food that contains a limited amount of saturated fat, trans fat, sugar, and sodium. Some researchers question whether the steps being taken by the FTC are meaningful, or if they go far enough (Kunkel, McKinley, & Wright, 2009). As of 2010, it is unknown if these standards and recommendations will be implemented. For more information on the proposed guidelines, visit www.foodpolitics.com/wp-content/uploads/working-group-recommendations.pdf.

second most plentiful ingredient is dextrose, a form of sugar, that sweetens the product to improve the flavor. Consumer understanding, knowledge, and concern with product ingredients can drive purchasing behavior. For example, consumers who are concerned with reducing sugar consumption may turn to a natural-style peanut butter that may not include the additional dextrose. Even in the case where there is a promotion or significant savings to be gained, consumers may still turn to the product with more desirable ingredients. Educational campaigns are needed to improve understanding of nutritional and healthy weight guidelines and how to meet them to aid consumers in making informed choices based on product labels.

Promotion refers to any publicity, advertising, or selling strategies that are associated with a product or service. At the point of purchase, promotions might include in-store marketing materials, like signs and coupons, along with free samples and product placement. It is widely recognized that targeted promotion using many communication channels is very common for many foods. For example, children's television programming frequently devotes a higher portion of advertising for child-oriented products such as sugary cereals, candy, or other snack items. At the retail point of purchase, targeted promotion is extended and intensified by the tangible presence of the product or service. For example, imagine that a popular fast-food company is promoting their children's meal with a particular movie character action figure. The company might saturate the television with commercial spots during children's television programs. This will, in turn, stimulate children to ask their parents for this restaurant even if a choice of restaurants is not given. At the restaurant, there may be large signs on the windows visible from the street. There may be more signs placed at a child's eye level, coordinating the television advertising with the point-of-purchase product availability. The product may then be purchased, satisfying not only immediate hunger, but also the psychological wanting of the product (i.e., wanting to eat without being physically hungry), increasing the likelihood of overweight. In addition, the toy action figure may be taken home for repeated play and repeated memory of the specific restaurant, leading to higher probability of repeated visits to the restaurant. These same coordinated promotion approaches can be used for healthier alternatives, but these are seldom seen.

Product placement not only refers to the shelf location of the product in a particular store, but also to the placement of a product in a particular area or neighborhood. The most desirable location for a product to be placed is in a highly visible spot (e.g., eye level) and close to the place of purchase (e.g., the cash register). Companies pay fees, called slotting fees, for the right to choose the shelf location of their products in stores and restaurants. These fees determine where the product is slotted. The belief is that people tend to select things that they see first, so products at eye level are more likely to be purchased. It is interesting to check this phenomenon out at the grocery store. For example, in the snack aisle, the chips that are the most popular and have the biggest marketing budget typically are located on the shelf that is easiest to see first—at eye level. This is particularly noticeable for products that are marketed to kids; they are often placed on shelves where kids are most likely to see them and prompt their parents to buy them. Products at the cash register are often items that are common impulse buys and are high in calories and contain few nutrients (e.g., candy and soda). Companies place products there so that consumers will deviate from their shopping list and purchase the item. This not only accomplishes the marketing goals of stimulating trial and purchase, but also allows companies to make more money because individual items purchased at the cash register are typically available in other store locations in larger quantities for a much lower price per unit. Consider that individual chewing gum packages at the check-out counter may cost as much as a third more than those found in a three pack in the candy aisle at the same supermarket.

Product placement also refers to the overall availability of items in stores or restaurants in a given area or neighborhood. Food companies often alter product distribution based on the sociodemographics of neighborhoods or market trends. For example, areas that have a higher proportion of a population under the age of 18 may have stores and restaurants that carry more products targeting children. In our previous fast-food restaurant example, this restaurant chain may build more restaurants in areas where there are more children, in an effort to serve more families with children, and in turn, sell more products. Impoverished areas often have fewer large supermarkets, and the small grocery stores and convenience stores that are more common in these areas tend to sell fewer healthful and nutritious foods at higher costs. Thus, living in socioeconomically deprived neighborhoods can mean access to fewer supermarkets but more convenience and small grocery stores than wealthier neighborhoods; that in turn may lead to obesogenic dietary habits (Chung, 1999; Moore & Diez Roux, 2006; Sooman, Macintyre, & Anderson, 1993; Wang, Kim, Gonzalez, MacLeod, & Winkleby, 2007; Zenk et al., 2005). These social injustices limit healthful food options and affect the diet of neighborhood residents.

Although it cannot be assumed that people purchase the majority of their food in their home neighborhood, people tend to make dietary choices based on the quality of food that is available and economical (Mooney, 1990; White, 1987). Residents in impoverished areas may have few individual capital resources, such as personal transportation, leading to greater reliance on nearby, albeit often limited, food sources (Cummins & Macintyre, 2006). Residents who rely on convenience stores, liquor stores, or small grocery stores may have a more limited and more expensive selection of healthful foods because larger supermarkets typically stock a wider variety of goods (Sooman et al., 1993; Wang et al., 2007). Like the lack of healthful food options, a deficiency of resources can lead to food insecurity and the excessive consumption of non-nutritious, processed foods (e.g., fast foods, packaged foods). Residents of deprived neighborhoods report eating fewer fruits and vegetables and more foods high in fat, even after adjusting for individual SES (Diez-Roux et al., 1999; Drewnowski & Darmon, 2005; Ellaway & Macintyre, 1996; Lee & Cubbin, 2002).

Pricing is the price of the product that the consumer actually pays. This may include not only the monetary price on the label and any price discounts, but exchangeable commodities such as time, attention, and energy. Price affects eating habits, and meeting dietary recommendations can be difficult because of the higher costs for many healthier foods combined with high cost of living (Jetter & Cassady, 2006; Poston & Foreyt, 1999). Foods that are high in sugar and oil are not only more filling and higher in calories but also typically less expensive to produce compared to more healthful foods that may be more nutritionally dense but less filling and lower in calories. Consumers with fixed budgets may find it appealing to buy larger quantities of less nutritious foods at lower prices. Other consumers may feel that the time to prepare nutritious food may be too costly; they may be willing to pay more for preprepared, packaged foods that may or may not be nutritionally similar.

Which of the four Ps is most important for retail point of purchase marketing, and why?

To compound the problem of placement discussed previously, it is often the case that stores found in impoverished neighborhoods may be more expensive than stores found in middle and higher income areas (Zhang & Wang, 2004). Differential pricing in stores found in impoverished neighborhoods suggests that small groceries, pharmacies, and convenience stores may be more expensive than supermarkets (Latham & Moffat, 2007; Sooman et al., 1993). Thus, differential pricing suggests that it is more costly to eat healthfully in impoverished neighborhoods, not only because of the price of the product itself but also because people who live in impoverished areas may need to travel further to get to stores and restaurants that have a variety of reasonably priced, nutritious, and delicious foods. Recent research has determined that large supermarkets and farmers' markets that rely on local foods are often the best places to find high-quality, lower-priced produce in U.S. cities, regardless of neighborhood SES (Lee, Heinrich, Medina, Regan, Reese-Smith, Jokura, & Maddock, 2010). Local efforts that help small-scale farmers get their products to local farmers' markets may help increase access to and consumption of more nutritious fresh foods. Capitalizing on regional strengths may be important for sustainable availability of a variety of healthful foods.

❑ Understand strategies used to promote trial and purchase of food at stores and restaurants.

❑ Distinguish among marketing, advertising, and branding and describe how each can be used to promote food at the retail point of purchase.

❑ Describe the four Ps and how they can influence purchase and consumption of food.

GETTING STARTED

Summary

The retail point of purchase plays an important role in the purchase and consumption decisions that consumers make every day. Marketing strategies tie the advertising to which consumers are exposed every day to the point of purchase where the product or service is actually acquired. Retail point of purchase is a powerful link back to other coordinated marketing and advertising. Public health promotion strategies often emphasize eating a variety of foods, but access to a variety of attractive, reasonably priced, easy-to-prepare foods may vary greatly from one neighborhood to the next. The retail point of purchase is an important venue for healthful food promotion in the attempt to prevent and treat the obesity epidemic; efforts that coordinate consumers, local farm bureaus, and merchants in the improvement of the point of purchase are needed.

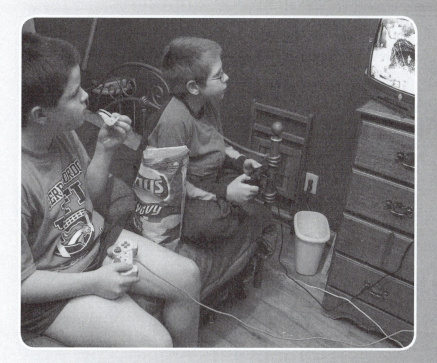

CHAPTER 14

Influence of Media and Technology

As technology and science continue to advance, the media becomes an increasingly influential factor in dietary habits and obesity. On average, Americans watch at least four hours of television a day and are also exposed to millions of food advertisements a year through the Internet, billboards, and other media sources (Bureau of Labor Statistics, 2009). While obesity levels continue to soar, the content and frequency of marketing deserves further examination. The impact of media is reflected by the success of numerous fast food restaurants and convenience stores and the hundreds of ways to purchase food. The substantial impact of media is not only evident by the success of these particular food microenvironments of the ecologic model of obesity but by the availability of fast food and prepackaged items in other microenvironments, particularly school and work. Schools and workplaces now have a plethora of food choices that include vending machines and fast-food restaurants within the facility. Food advertisements are on billboards and points of purchase, and they are now seen on televisions, computers, and MP3 players and phones. As technological innovation continues to advance, particularly among mobile media, food advertisements can be viewed in and across almost any microenvironment, making them more influential and accessible than ever.

One reason why food advertising is such a successful endeavor is the appetizing imagery used in marketing. Food images can serve as a hunger stimulus by triggering individual biological responses. This chapter discusses the implications of these visual stimuli and the increasing number of sources that provide them.

Biological Responses to Food Images

It is no surprise that pictures of appealing food make viewers feel hungry or make them believe that they are. Studies continue to conclude that visual representations of appetizing foods stimulate biological responses within the brain (Francis et al., 1999; Simmons, Martin, & Barsalou, 2005). The brain's gustatory processing regions store visual information, produce responses to taste, and distribute the information for later use with pictures of food. The brain's gustatory processing areas are located on the anterior insula on the insular lobe and the frontal operculum on the inferior frontal gyrus of the frontal lobe and the left orbitofrontal cortex. Gustatory processing processes can all occur subconsciously, without intentionality (Simmons et al., 2005).

Gustatory processing region = the area of the brain that processes flavors and tastes.

Among the millions of food and beverage advertisements in America, few people are aware of the impact of just one look at a picture of food. As an onlooker glances at an image of food, visual properties of the object become a part of a distributed circuit of information sent to and across modality-specific areas of the brain (Martin, 2001; Martin & Chao, 2001; Thompson-Schill, 2003). Images of food can activate areas of the brain that are very close to areas that become stimulated when people actually eat food. This proximity suggests that food images can automatically activate gustatory areas and produce theoretical inferences about their tastes. The object is then processed and association areas retain information for later use. This often occurs unknowingly to the observer (Simmons et al., 2005).

People are exposed to food advertisements on billboards as they travel to and from work. At work, they connect to the Internet where they are exposed to all sorts of food advertisements. At home, many view food commercials during their favorite television programs. Most people are constantly bombarded with visual stimulation that is stored for later use; this can have serious implications since it can lead to desires to overeat unhealthful food, which in turn contributes to obesity and its resulting adverse health conditions.

Sometimes even simply thinking about food, which often follows a visual or auditory prompt, can activate areas of the brain that process taste and taste reward (Simmons et al., 2005). Food images followed by the location of the food also create significant gustatory stimulation. One study done by Simmons suggests that a food picture followed by the food's location or source (i.e., restaurant) produces taste inferences (Simmons et al., 2005). It isn't surprising, then, that advertisers create ads for food that are followed by the food's location or producer. Placement, timing, and sequence have all become effective marketing strategies for food marketers.

Television Advertising and Children

Most Americans watch several hours of television each night and are bombarded by commercials (Holmes, 2008). But Americans are not alone in their television habits, despite the health detriments associated with excessive viewing. Researchers in Australia found that television viewing time was associated with increased risk of all-cause mortality and cardiovascular disease mortality (Dunstan et al., 2010). As television viewing time increases, so does commercial viewing.

Television advertisements are now a multimillion-dollar method of promoting the latest food product or beverage. The accessibility of a television and time to watch is also an issue for many children. Recent research suggests that children are now watching more television than ever with black and Latino children watching more television than white children (Dennison, Erb, & Jenkins, 2002; Viner & Cole, 2005). This is a public health concern because watching television typically decreases physical activity and increases the likelihood of poor dietary habits and child overweight and obesity (Gable, Chang, & Krull, 2007). For example, each additional hour of television that 5-year-olds watch on weekends increases their risk of adult obesity by 7% (Viner & Cole, 2005). Furthermore, a recent study from the American Academy of Pediatrics found that children who spend the most time watching television have higher blood pressure, regardless of body composition, compared to those who watch very little or no television (Martinez-Gomez, Tucker, Heelan, Welk, & Eisenmann, 2009). Watching television as a child can also predict future dietary habits. One recent study looked at two groups of adolescents (middle school and high school) and found that heavy television viewers reported lower fruit and vegetable intakes five years later.

Televisions are often a substitute family member for a busy household, regardless of people's awareness of the increased health risks associated with excessive exposure. Low socioeconomic status (SES) and income levels have been linked to increased television viewing and decreased physical activity (Bennett et al., 2006; Multimedia Audiences Summary, 2003). Recent research has shown that children who watch more television are more likely to be overweight or obese and children from low-income families who have a television in their room have an even higher risk of being overweight (Burdette & Whitaker, 2005; Dennison et al., 2002). Another alarming finding suggested that children from families who watch television during meals eat more meat, pizza, salty snacks, and soda than children who do not watch television during family meals (Coon, Goldberg, Rogers, & Tucker, 2001).

Although not every family owns a computer or has Internet access at home, televisions are prevalent in American households. As more families become two-working-parent households, more children come home to empty houses, resulting in television watching that is unsupervised and excessive. Parents who are absent or are busy when at home often rely on the television to provide stimulation, comfort, and entertainment (Dennison et al., 2002). As children view more television, they are also exposed to more commercials. Food advertising accounts for nearly half of these commercials, the vast majority of which are for energy dense foods of poor nutritional content (Powell, Szczypka,

Implementing Policy

TV Turnoff Week

Many communities have begun implementing TV Turnoff Week campaigns in order to reduce the amount of television watched. Turning off the TV for a week increases time that might be used for more physically active recreational activities and reduces exposure to advertisements for foods high in fat, sugar, and sodium. Less extreme reduction activities include removing televisions from bedrooms, turning off the television during meals, and budgeting viewing time to watch specific shows. The less time children spend watching TV or playing video games, the less weight they gain over time. Studies suggest that this relationship may be driven more by reduced consumption than increased energy expenditure (Epstein et al., 2008), possibly reflecting the cessation of overeating while watching TV or reduced susceptibility to consuming heavily marketed, energy-dense foods.

Chaloupka, & Braunschweig, 2007; Stitt & Kunkel, 2008). Not surprisingly, one study found that watching food commercials cued a significantly higher commercial recall in an after-movie questionnaire for young children. The children were also allowed to freely snack while watching the commercials. Boys ate more snack foods when watching the food commercials than neutral commercials (although girls ate slightly less). Further, since the snack food was a non-advertised food brand, the increased caloric consumption was not a function of brand recognition (Anschutz, Engels, & Van Strien, 2009). The net result is an increased risk for many lifelong adverse health consequences.

Television commercials are the most prominent form of marketing in the home, with food advertisements heavily represented. These food advertisements use publicly recognizable figures, branding, and popular cartoon, television, and movie characters in order to attract a child's attention (Coon et al., 2001). These tactics create an exciting, pleasurable experience for the viewer. Most food television commercials equate food with fun and pleasure, creating an even stronger ploy to persuade viewers to purchase and consume the product (Connor, 2006).

Public figures, ranging from athletes to musicians, are often a frequent component of television advertisements. Fast-food and beverage companies often use music and dance personalities to display their latest creation. Jessica and Ashlee Simpson, two pop music artists, have collaborated to sell Pizza Hut products, while other singers, like Britney Spears and Beyoncé, have advertised for Pepsi. Celebrity influence is a high priority for food producers, and many large corporations choose to have celebrities represent their products. The image of a popular personality can increase sales and marketability tremendously. In contrast, public figures are rarely involved with alcohol and drug-related advertisements, shying away from potentially controversial advertisements. Instead music, television, movie, and athletic personalities choose to attach their characters to safer products like fast food or soft drinks even though overconsumption of processed and fattening foods can lead to life-threatening conditions.

Food corporations have a variety of methods to target children and adolescents based on their preferences and the current culture. Branding can begin as early as preschool (Connor, 2006). Branding is an advertising tactic designed to establish product familiarity and to form positive associations with a product or company name. The goal of branding for young children is to produce recognition of company names and products, increasing the likelihood of future use as an adult. Branding can be created through a memorable musical theme or sequence of events. Often children can remember a commercial's song or tune which can later trigger recollection of the product. The Kaiser Family Foundation surveyed parents of children six years old and younger and found that, on an average day, over half of the children under age two watch television even though the American Academy of Pediatrics does not recommend television viewing for children two years of age and younger (Connor, 2006; Rideout, Hamel, & Kaiser Family Foundation, 2006). To capture the attention of these young children, food producers often use cartoon, movie, and TV characters. Ronald McDonald, representing McDonald's, and the Trix Rabbit are licensed characters that can assist in the branding process. Often these characters are cross-referenced and used in other food marketing corporation strategies. Examples of these are Teletubby Happy Meals and popular Disney characters that are used to promote fast food.

As described previously, the stimulation of gustatory processes from food pictures and the frequency of commercials and images are important among food promoters of children's programming. Children's television is regularly bombarded with food and beverage advertisements, with some programs being openly supported by these companies. Nickelodeon's Nick Jr. block draws up to one million viewers ages two to five each weekday and is supported openly by advertisements (Connor, 2006). Other channels like the Disney Channel and Public Broadcasting Service (PBS) are commercial free, but they still rely on corporate sponsors who supply underwriting credits. The high frequency of food-related commercials cannot be denied. A recent study found that in 96 half-hour blocks of preschool programming, Nickelodeon, the Disney Channel, and PBS had a total of 130 food-related advertisements. The majority of the advertisements aimed at children were for fast food and sweetened cereals (Connor, 2006).

Regardless of whether children have access to television at home, many view televised advertisements at school. Channel One, a popular educational program in American middle and high schools, airs 2 minutes of commercials with every 10 minutes of current-events programming (Strasburger, 2006). Even if children are not exposed to food advertisements within the home, they will more than likely see hundreds of commercials in school.

A typical child or adolescent sees about 40,000 television advertisements a year despite the Children's Television Act of 1990. This law limits advertising on children's programming to 10.5 minutes per hour on weekends and 12 minutes per hour on weekdays (Strasburger, 2006). Along with the high amount of food and beverage promotion, nutritional misinformation can often result (American Dietetic Association, 2006). Studies have shown that high-fat and high-sugar foods like candy, soft drinks, convenience and fast foods are most frequently advertised (Harrison & Marske, 2005; Powell et al., 2007). Furthermore, children who view junk food ads report a lower liking of healthful foods (Dixon, Scully, Wakefield, White, & Crawford, 2007).

Researchers continue to report that television food advertising increases children's preferences for the advertised foods and their requests for those foods (Harris, Brownell, & Bargh, 2009). One study estimated the effects of television fast-food restaurant advertising on the childhood obesity epidemic and found that banning fast-food restaurant advertising would reduce the number of overweight children ages 3 to 11 in a fixed population by 18% and would reduce the number of overweight adolescents ages 12 to 18 by 14%. The effects of television advertising on childhood obesity cannot be denied (Chou, Rashad, & Grossman, 2008).

With the known negative effects of television viewing and advertisements on children, researchers have begun extensive studies of new approaches for a better understanding of how food marketing affects young people. For example, the newly developed food marketing defense model presents four necessary conditions to effectively counter harmful food marketing practices: awareness, understanding, ability, and motivation to resist (Harris et al., 2009). Food marketing defense models like these are often used to create media literacy education materials. Media literacy education and methods used to dispute unsound nutrition information are discussed later in the chapter.

The implications of children's excessive television exposure are apparent during adolescence. Adolescents are increasingly more overweight and sedentary, leading to health problems in their youth and later adulthood (Ogden, Carroll, & Flegal, 2008). Overweight adolescents have more weight struggles, willpower issues, and family problems compared to those of normal weight (Glessner, Hoover, & Halzlett, 2006). In particular, adolescent girls may experience body image pressures perpetuated by media-generated images because both television commercials and programs often present young, thin, attractive people. The heavy reliance on television as entertainment may contribute to serious health problems such as obesity for today's youth.

Internet Advertising

Although television may be the most prominent form of media exposure, with computer use in the home rising, the Internet is quickly gaining ground (Weber, Story, & Harnack, 2006). Internet food and beverage advertising has emerged as an entirely new marketing tool. Pop-up advertisements, attractive links, and games have all surfaced on popular Web sites. A mouth-watering picture of a cookie and a thirst-quenching soda can now be viewed with the click of a mouse on thousands of sites. Many Web sites also have interactive games and challenges that are sponsored by large food and beverage companies.

Like television, Internet advertisers intentionally target children and adolescents. *Advergaming,* entertainment in which the advertised product is part of the game, and other interactive areas are common ploys for a child's attention (Weber et al., 2006). One study found that the Web sites of over half of the top five selling brands in eight food and beverage

> Advergaming = advertising + gaming = the practice of using a video game to advertise a product.

categories contained advergaming and cartoon characters (Weber et al., 2006). Both children and adolescents are frequently targeted with banners, games, and catalogs. Another study evaluated ten popular children's Web sites and found food advertisements on seven of them. These advertisements primarily promoted candy, cereal, fast-food restaurants, and snacks (Alvy & Calvert, 2008). It is clear that, in general, this type of advertising is not consistent with a healthful diet.

Despite the increase in Internet sales, there remains a lack of regulation for food and beverage marketing that targets children. Although the Children's Online Privacy Protection Act of 1998 prohibits sites from knowingly collecting information from children younger than 13 years of age, lack of parental supervision can allow a child to supply personal information that can eventually be harmful. When this information is supplied, marketers are able to compile it for sale to third parties, allowing complete strangers to use the information to contact children for various reasons including the promotion of energy-dense food.

Billboard Advertising

Billboard advertising has been a successful approach for food and beverage marketers. The average American commuting to work probably encounters at least one billboard or sign on route. Motor vehicles have even become traveling billboard advertisements as large trucks, buses, and cars promote products and services. Chances are that if you are traveling on a major highway or busy road, you will come across an appetizing image, information regarding food and beverages, or a company that markets food and beverages.

As described earlier, the gustatory processing regions remember these types of images and store them for later use. Simmons found that viewing food images for just two seconds activates the gustatory cortex, a region of the brain that represents the taste of food (Simmons et al., 2005). After viewing several food advertisement billboards each day, the brain remembers the picture and actually infers a taste. Findings such as these reinforce the major impact of advertising on promoting obesity.

Sport Sponsorships

Sport sponsorship has also become a profitable method of food and beverage advertising. Many fans equate athletics with money, success, and fame, along with exceptional health. Perceptions of physical activity and well-being are attractive to most people; as a result, products that are linked with the sport or physical activity through sponsorship often benefit from this association.

Although sport participation itself is usually health promoting, studies suggest that most sport sponsorships are associated with unhealthy food—energy-dense products high in calories or containing empty calories. Alcohol, processed foods, and high sugar foods are often coupled with athletics at the club, regional, and national levels. It is not unusual to see a popular sporting event being sponsored by a beverage or fast-food company. Maher and colleagues found that sport sponsorships were associated with unhealthy foods more than twice as often as healthy foods. Their study suggested that the sponsorships of popular sports for young people are predominately unhealthy and should require government review and possible future regulation (Maher, Wilson, Signal, & Thomson, 2006).

Media Intervention Strategies

Although the majority of food advertising and media promote unhealthy foods and beverages, there also have been influential media outlets for health. School and community campaigns have increased their health education strategies, such as launching public health interventions to increase information and providing tools for parents and teachers, despite unhealthy food marketing. Some of these are discussed in chapter 9. We outline some other examples in the following sections.

Dietary Habits

A public health intervention, according to the National Institute for Health and Clinical Excellence, is any advice, service, or support that helps reduce people's risk of developing a chronic disease or condition or helps to promote a healthy lifestyle (National Institute for Health and Clinical Excellence, 2009). The MyPyramid for Kids is an example of a public health intervention (figure 14.1). Point-of-purchase materials in the cafeteria and classroom have included brochures and newsletters that use the pyramid to inform adults on the food they and their children are consuming. These strategies have been shown to increase children's knowledge and intake of fruits and vegetables (Anderson et al., 2005).

Due to the rise of obesity in more urban, low-income, and minority areas, citywide media interventions have become an accepted means of educating the public domain. Community campaigns have demonstrated effectiveness through radio, television advertising, and bus and streetcar signage. The National 5 a Day campaign was a countrywide attempt to educate citizens on the importance of consuming fruits and vegetables and motivate more people to consume them regularly. Now called Fruits and Veggies Matter, the media campaign and point-of-purchase program are designed to increase the consumption of a variety of fruits and vegetables based on one's age and sex (CDC, 2009). Another community-based campaign promoted consumption of low-fat milk through paid advertising and public relations movements. As a result, citizens increased both low-fat and overall milk consumption (Reger, Wootan, Booth-Butterfield, & Smith, 1998).

Physical Activity

Along with dietary intervention movements, community campaigns promoting physical activity are also emerging. To promote physical activity, in 2002 the Center of Disease Control and Prevention launched the multiethnic VERB campaign

What are some media intervention strategies that organizations (e.g., schools, the CDC) can use to educate and inform children and adolescents of healthful activities?

using paid advertisements, school and community promotions, and Internet activities. Huhman found that, as a result of the campaign, children's awareness

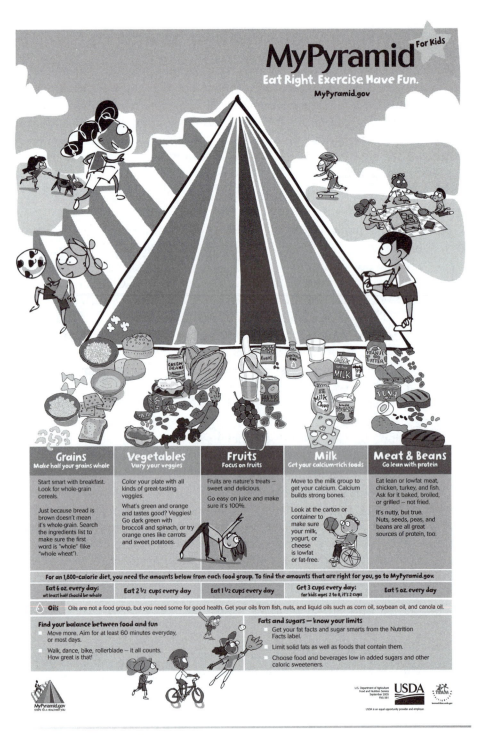

FIGURE 14.1 MyPyramid for Kids.

U.S. Department of Agriculture

and self-reported physical activity increased (Huhman et al., 2005). Children's programming has also begun to feature children and celebrities engaging in physical activity. In particular, the Children's Television Network has done extensive work to promote healthful eating and physical activity. The network uses popular television characters engaging in physical activities and making choices to eat fruits and vegetables over less nutritious choices (Children's TV Network, 2009).

Technological Innovations

In addition to point-of-purchase materials and national and community-based campaigns, technological innovations have become a popular and possibly more efficient media intervention strategy. Technology is increasing at a more rapid pace than is imaginable. We live in a world where we have constant, instant access to information on a vast array of topics, can reach our family and friends wherever we go, and are constantly fascinated by the latest innovations. People of all walks of life use the Internet daily, and instant translation computer programs allow for communication among people who speak different languages from very different cultures.

Social networking Internet programs have become wildly popular, allowing people to share information, pictures, and events with large numbers of friends or colleagues. Sites such as Facebook and LinkedIn grow measurably every day. These kinds of social networks can be used to transmit information about obesity and the environment and to find others with common goals for healthful living.

Immersive virtual environments have also gained in popularity, in particular with education and gaming communities. Virtual environments like World of Warcraft or Second Life allow users to create an avatar that they operate from their computer keyboard. In these virtual environments, people can play games with other users, meet and talk with others about common interests, and develop lifelong friendships. These communities also allow educators to provide course content without the burden of geographic proximity. Some kinds of learning experiences are particularly suited to virtual environments. For example, the National Institutes of Health has developed a giant arterial vessel that one's avatar can explore to learn more about heart disease and stroke. The Texas Obesity Research Center has launched an International Health Challenge that explores the utility of virtual worlds in innovative health interventions.

Goods and services are also widely connected via technology. Telecommuting has made traveling to work an archaic concept for some industries. Shopping online for a range of products from food to clothes to fitness equipment is de rigueur for many. Online coaches and training programs may help computer users get out into the world and move more. Mapping programs help walkers and runners map routes for physical activity to help users meet specific training goals (for instance, run hills), find an inspiring environment, or avoid unsafe areas. The Rails-to-Trails Conservancy has launched TrailLink .com, where users can find old rail lines that have been converted to bicycle or pedestrian trails. Users can link these trails to local bicycle routes and other trails on the Web site for free (Rails-to-Trails Conservancy, n.d.).

At the same time that Internet-based innovations are enjoyed and used by many, these kinds of technologies may also contribute to obesity by inspiring sedentary behavior. Rather than walking to the store, one can simply shop online. Rather than visiting neighbors in the neighborhood, one can simply see them on a social networking site. There are advantages and disadvantages to these innovations, and careful awareness and planning are needed to capitalize on technology without falling prey to it.

Technological innovation is able to connect people and information now more easily than ever, but resources are needed to set up networks and train people on how to use them effectively. Computerized patient records—important for coordinated wellness planning across many health professionals—are already possible, yet only slowly being instituted. Computerized patient records have the power to streamline patient care and reduce medical errors; however, the computerized system requires additional training and access to secure computer stations. Many complex computer simulations and projections for community designers and policy makers are available, but it is unclear whether they are widely used and whether the programs include parameters focused on improving health.

Another powerful implication of mobile technology is individual monitoring and telemetry. With handheld technology, it is possible to transmit information about physical activity, active transportation routes, speed, and medium (e.g., walk versus bike) as well as information about where, when, what, and how much is eaten to a master server where data can be uploaded. Health care providers have the power to monitor and provide feedback for their patients who need more physical activity or improved dietary habits to meet recommendations or lose weight.

Virtual environments, social networking, the exchange of goods and services, and individual monitoring can all be effective and efficient media intervention strategies to prevent and treat obesity. With technological innovation, most of these tasks can even be accomplished using handheld, mobile technology. Because so many people have Internet access and use some form of mobile technology, these media intervention strategies could be successful ways to educate and monitor users. When employing these innovations, there are advantages and disadvantages that should be considered, and more study is needed to clarify the intervention strategies that are most effective for various populations.

What can parents do to educate their children about healthy nutrition and physical activity to counteract the unhealthy messages they're exposed to on TV, the Internet, and the radio?

Media Literacy Education

As science and technology create new processed foods and additives, misinformation about nutrition has surfaced across the nation. Low-carbohydrate diets and "miracle" foods and drinks promise to melt excess weight without exercise. To counter

> Media literacy education = teaching strategies and tools to analyze, evaluate, and create media messages.

this marketing, the American Dietetic Association encourages proper nutrition education through nationally credentialed professionals. Successful nutrition communication includes simple yet informative content that helps consumers identify misinformation on food and nutrition.

Communities are also teaching citizens to become more media literate in order to prevent the proliferation of misinformation in the public domain. Media literacy education is a tool that teaches children and adults how to recognize, deconstruct, and evaluate media messages and create their own ideas (Division of Community Health, Nutrition Training Institute, 2005). Media literacy education in communities is becoming a recognized prevention tool to counteract the misinformation food and beverage companies often promote. Such training attempts to decrease media influence and obesity rates through educating health and wellness educators, nurses, physicians, and teachers on how to distinguish fact from fiction.

❏ Describe the biologic response and appetite-stimulation power of media images.
❏ Understand the influence of the television on health habits and obesity.
❏ Describe the role that the Internet plays in influencing obesity.
❏ Describe other forms of media that may contribute to obesity.
❏ Identify technological advancements that may serve in the pursuit of better coordination.

GETTING STARTED

Summary

As obesity continues to affect the health of our nation, health professionals and citizens should not underestimate the influence of the widespread media. Food and beverage marketers now have a plethora of sources to promote their products. Gone are the days of hearsay's influence because television, Internet, billboards, point-of-purchase materials, and sponsorships dominate the public domain. While the prevalence of media exposure increases, the public must retain control of content and exposure to messages through health interventions and media literacy education. Technological innovations like online social networking, immersive virtual environments, and online goods and service exchanges can be an effective way to intervene, but advantages and disadvantages must be considered. Although adults might have the personal responsibility to properly educate themselves on nutrition information, attention should shift to the obesity epidemic of today's children. Whether it's a commercial for the latest cereal with a new toy or a new game on the Internet sponsored by a soft drink company, combating the message doesn't change: Children must be taught sound nutrition information. It is only when media, policy makers, industry, educators, and parents work together that obesity among children will be reversed.

EPILOGUE

If there is one thing that readers might take away from this book, it's that the environments that surround us every day have endless layers of complexity, and the layers are all interrelated. These interrelationships point to an even greater complexity; changing any one thing may have both expected and unexpected consequences that may be good or bad, or both, or neither. Nevertheless, better coordination of strategies to prevent and reduce obesity is desperately needed. This is not a job for any one person or even one country; rather, a global strategy that brings together many partners representing nations, corporations, scientists, practitioners, policy makers, health care providers, and the public is needed.

The World Health Organization serves as the international agency for coordinating efforts related to health; in fact, there are already efforts underway to reduce obesity and reverse the obesogenic environment. However, it is unclear whether these efforts are sufficient in scope and representation to have more than a negligible effect. Dr. James Hill, a well-known scientist in obesity research, tells us that our generation will be judged by the way it handles the current obesity pandemic. At our current trajectory, we will be judged as failures. Obesity, and our obesogenic environment, are not as glamorous as some diseases, and because of the slow and chronic nature of the disease, sometimes it is easy to ignore its progression.

In the time it has taken to write this book, the world has changed, but the population continues to increase in girth. There is no apparent end in sight to the obesogenesis of our society. It is a most vexing problem. We like to believe that just one person with courage and persistence can make a difference, but it is unclear now whether this is sufficient. We encourage all readers to talk to a friend about the things learned in this book. If you agree with these premises, read more about the issues in the daily newspaper, or online, or wherever you can find information. If you disagree with us, find evidence that supports your position, and tell us about it. We really believe that science and health practitioners know enough to change the world—the evidence exists already, so now it's your turn to take action. Tell your friends, lobby your policy makers, join a volunteer organization, and work for the cause. You are the future, and we hope you make it a healthier one for everyone!

REFERENCES

Chapter 1

Bronfenbrenner, U. (1977). Toward an experimental ecology of human development. *American Psychologist, 32*, 513-531.

Bronfenbrenner, U. (1979). *The ecology of human development: Experiments by nature and design.* Cambridge, MA: Havard University Press.

Buscher, L.A., Martin, K.A., & Crocker, S. (2001). Point-of-purchase messages framed in terms of cost, convenience, taste, and energy improve healthful snack selection in a college foodservice setting. *Journal of American Dietetic Association, 101*(8), 909-913.

Centers for Disease Control and Prevention & National Center for Injury Prevention and Control. (2008). WISQARS Leading Causes of Death Reports, 1999 – 2005. Retrieved from http://webapp.cdc.gov/sasweb/ncipc/leadcaus10.html

Chen, A.H., Sallis, J.F., Castro, C.M., Lee, R.E., Hickmann, S.A., William, C., & Martin, J.E. (1998). A home-based behavioral intervention to promote walking in sedentary ethnic minority women: Project WALK. *Womens Health, 4*(1), 19-39.

Collins, R., Lee, R.E., Albright, C.L., & King, A.C. (2004). Ready to be physically active? The effects of a course preparing low-income multiethnic women to be more physically active. *Health Educ Behav, 31*(1), 47-64.

Costa, D.L., & Steckel, R.H. (1997). Long-term trends in health, welfare, and economics growth in the United States. In R. Floud and R.H. Steckel (Eds.), *Health and welfare during industrialization.* Chicago: University of Chicago Press.

Cubbin, C., & Winkleby, M.A. (2005). Protective and harmful effects of neighborhood-level deprivation on individual-level health knowledge, behavior, and risk of coronary heart disease. *American Journal of Epidemiology 162*(6), 559-568.

Dishman, R.K. (1994). The measurement conundrum in exercise adherence research. *Medicine and Science Sports Exercise, 26*(11), 1382-1390.

Dishman, R.K., & Buckworth, J. (1996). Increasing physical activity: A quantitative synthesis. *Med Sci Sports Exerc, 28*(6), 706-719.

Eyler, A.A., Brownson, R.C., Bacak, S.J., & Housemann, R.A. (2003). The epidemiology of walking for physical activity in the United States. *Med Sci Sports Exerc, 35*(9), 1529-1536.

Flegal, K.M., Carroll, M.D., Ogden, C.L., & Johnson, C.L. (2002). Prevalence and trends in obesity among U.S. adults, 1999-2000. *JAMA, 288*(14), 1723-1727.

Giles-Corti, B., & Donovan, R.J. (2003). Relative influences of individual, social environmental, and physical environmental correlates of walking. *Am J Public Health, 93*(9), 1583-1589.

Guyer, B., Freedman, M.A., Strobino, D.M., & Sondik, E.J. (2000). Annual summary of vital statistics: Trends in the health of Americans during the 20th century. *Pediatrics, 106*(6), 1307-1317.

Horgen, K.B., & Brownell, K.D. (2002). Comparison of price change and health message interventions in promoting healthy food choices. *Health Psychol, 21*(5), 505-512.

Hunt, M.K., Lefebvre, R.C., Hixson, M.L., Banspach, S.W., Assaf, A.R., & Carleton, R.A. (1990). Pawtucket Heart Health Program point-of-purchase nutrition education program in supermarkets. *Am J Public Health, 80*(6), 730-732.

Klem, M.L., Wing, R.R., Lang, W., McGuire, M.T., & Hill, J.O. (2000). Does weight loss maintenance become easier over time? *Obes Res, 8*(6), 438-444.

Lalonde, M. (1974). *A new perspective on the health of Canadians. A working document.* Ottawa: Government of Canada.

Lee, R.E., & Cubbin, C. (2009). Striding toward social justice: The ecologic milieu of physical activity. *Exerc Sport Sci Rev, 37*(1), 10-17.

McLeroy, K.R., Bibeau, D., Steckler, A., & Glanz, K. (1988). An ecological perspective on health promotion programs. *Health Educ Q, 15*(4), 351-377.

Mokdad, A.H., Marks, J.S., Stroup, D.F., & Gerberding, J.L. (2004). Actual causes of death in the United States, 2000. *JAMA, 291*(10), 1238-1245.

Mooney, C. (1990). Cost and availability of healthy food choices in a London health district. *J Hum Nutr Diet, 3*(2), 111-120.

Morland, K., Wing, S., & Diez Roux, A. (2002). The contextual effect of the local food environment on residents' diets: The atherosclerosis risk in communities study. *Am J Public Health, 92*(11), 1761-1767.

Morland, K., Wing, S., Diez Roux, A., & Poole, C. (2002). Neighborhood characteristics associated with the location of food stores and food service places. *Am J Prev Med, 22*(1), 23-29.

Ogden, C.L., Carroll, M.D., Curtin, L.R., McDowell, M.A., Tabak, C.J., & Flegal, K.M. (2006). Prevalence of overweight and obesity in the United States, 1999-2004. *JAMA, 295*(13), 1549-1555.

Ogden, C.L., Carroll, M.D., & Flegal, K.M. (2008). High body mass index for age among U.S. children and adolescents, 2003-2006. *JAMA, 299*(20), 2401-2405.

Ogden, C.L., Flegal, K.M., Carroll, M.D., & Johnson, C.L. (2002). Prevalence and trends in overweight among U.S. children and adolescents 1999-2000. *JAMA, 288*(14), 1728-1732.

Ono, T., Guthold, R., & Strong, K. (2005). WHO Global comparable estimates infobase. Geneva, Switzerland: World Health Organization. Retrieved from https://apps.who.int/infobase/Index.aspx

Poston, W.S., Haddock, C.K., Olvera, N.E., Suminski, R.R., Reeves, R.S., Dunn, J.K., Hanis, C.L., & Foreyt, J.P. (2001). Evaluation of a culturally appropriate intervention to increase physical activity. *Am J Health Behav, 25*(4), 396-406.

Regan, G., Lee, R.E., Booth, K., & Reese-Smith, J. (2006). Obesogenic influences in public housing: A mixed-method analysis. *American Journal of Health Promotion, 20*(4), 282-290.

Resnicow, K., Jackson, A., Braithwaite, R., DiIorio, C., Blisset, D., Rahotep, S., & Periasamy, S. (2002). Healthy body/healthy spirit: A church-based nutrition and physical activity intervention. *Health Educ Res, 17*(5), 562-573.

Sallis, J.F., Bauman, A., & Pratt, M. (1998). Environmental and policy interventions to promote physical activity. *Am J Prev Med, 15*(4), 379-397.

Sallis, J.F., & Owen, N. (1997). *Ecological models.* (2nd ed.). San Francisco: Jossy-Bass.

Spence, J.C., & Lee, R.E. (2003). Toward a comprehensive model of physical activity. *Psychol Sport Exerc, 4*(1), 7-24.

Wang Y., & Lobstein, T. (2006). Worldwide trends in childhood overweight and obesity. *Int J Pediatr Obes, 1*(1), 11-25.

Chapter 2

American Association of Retired Persons. (2009). Activity calculator. Retreived from www.aarp.org/health/healthyliving/activity_calculator

American College of Sports Medicine. (2006). Lessons in youth activity. Retrieved from www.acsm.org/AM/Template.cfm?Section=ACSM_News_Releases&CONTENTID=5364&TEMPLATE=/CM/ContentDisplay.cfm

American College of Sports Medicine and the American Heart Association. (2007). Guidelines for healthy adults under age 65. Retrieved from www.acsm.org/AM/Template.cfm?Section=Home_Page&TEMPLATE=CM/HTMLDisplay.cfm&CONTENTID=7764#Under_65

American Heart Association. (2010). Physical activity. Retrieved from www.americanheart.org/presenter.jhtml?identifier=4563

Bahr, D.B., Browning, R.C., Wyatt, H.R., & Hill, J.O. (2009). Exploiting social networks to mitigate the obesity epidemic. *Obesity (Silver Spring), 17*(4), 723-728.

Baum, C.L., 2nd, & Ford, W.F. (2004). The wage effects of obesity: A longitudinal study. *Health Econ, 13*(9), 885-899.

Cawley, J. (2000). An instrumental variables approach to measuring the effect of body weight on employment disability. *Health Serv Res, 35*(5 Pt 2), 1159-1179.

Cawley, J. (2004). The impact of obesity on wages. *Journal of Human Resources, 39*(2), 452-474.

Centers for Disease Control and Prevention. (2008). Behavioral Risk Factor Surveillance System annual survey data. Retrieved from www.cdc.gov/brfss/technical_infodata/surveydata/2008.htm

Centers for Disease Control and Prevention. (2010). How much physical activity do children need? Retrieved from www.cdc.gov/physicalactivity/everyone/guidelines/children.html

Finkelstein, E. A., Fiebelkorn, I. C., & Wang, G. (2003). National medical spending attributable to overweight and obesity: How much, and who's paying? *Health Aff (Millwood), Suppl Web Exclusives*, W3-219-226.

Forbes, G.B. (1999). Longitudinal changes in adult fat-free mass: Influence of body weight. *Am J Clin Nutr, 70*(6), 1025-1031.

Gibbs, W.W. (1996). Gaining on fat. *Sci Am, 275*(2), 88-94.

Himmelstein, D.U., Warren, E., Thorne, D., & Woolhandler, S. (2005). Illness and injury as contributors to bankruptcy. *Health Aff (Millwood), Suppl Web Exclusives*, W5-63-W65-73.

Institute of Medicine of the National Academies of Science. (2002). Dietary reference intakes for energy, carbohydrate, fiber, fat, fatty acids, cholesterol, protein, and amino acids. Washington, D.C.: National Academies Press.

Justus, M., Ryan, K., Rockenbach, J., Katterapalli, C., & Card-Higginson, P. (2007). Lessons learned while implementing a legislated school policy: Body mass index assessments among Arkansas's public school students. *J Sch Health, 77*(10), 706-713.

Kannel, W.B., D'Agostino, R.B., & Cobb, J.L. (1996). Effect of weight on cardiovascular disease. *Am J Clin Nutr, 63*(3 Suppl), 419S-422S.

Leade Health. (2006). White paper: Employee obesity is number one factor in productivity loss. Retrieved from www.insurancenewsnet.com/article.asp?a=featured_pr&id=60775

Lee, R.E. (2009). Personal Communication. Washington D.C.

Misra, A., & Khurana, L. (2008). Obesity and the metabolic syndrome in developing countries. *J Clin Endocrinol Metab, 93*(11 Suppl 1), S9-30.

Moore, S., Hall, J., Harper, S., & Lynch, J.W. (2010). Global and national socioeconomic disparities in obesity, overweight, and underweight status. *Journal of Obesity, 2010.*[epub 8/20/2010]

Morris, S. (2007). The impact of obesity on employment. *Labour Economics, 14*(3), 413-433.

Nagourney, R.A. (2000, November 28). Bigger needles for better vaccinations. *New York Times.*

National Heart, Lung, and Blood Institute of the National Institutes of Health. (1998). *Clinical guidelines on the identification, evaluation, and treatment of overweight and obesity: The evidence report.* Washington, D.C.: U.S. Government Press.

Nifong, T.P., & Gerhard, G.S. (1999). Physical determinants of line pressures during apheresis. *Transfus Sci, 20*(3), 167-173.

Ogden, C.L., Carroll, M.D., Curtin, L.R., McDowell, M.A., Tabak, C.J., & Flegal, K.M. (2006). Prevalence of overweight and obesity in the United States, 1999-2004. *JAMA, 295*(13), 1549-1555.

Ogden, C.L., Carroll, M.D., McDowell, M.A., & Flegal, K.M. (2007). Obesity among adults in the United States: No statistically significant change since 2003-2004. *NCHS Data Brief* (1), 1-8.

Patton, P. (1999, September 23). America's ever-bigger bottoms bedeviling seating planners. *Miami Herald.* Retrieved from www.lakofsky.com/articles/biggerbottoms.html

Phillips, D. (2003, September 20). JetBlue apologizes for use of passenger records. *Washington Post.* Retrieved from www.washingtonpost.com

Pinot de Moira, A., Power, C., & Li, L. (2010). Changing influences on childhood obesity: A study of 2 generations of the 1958 British birth cohort. *Am J Epidemiol, 171*(12), 1289-1298.

Puhl, R.M., & Heuer, C.A. (2009). The stigma of obesity: A review and update. *Obesity (Silver Spring), 17*(5), 941-964.

Satcher, D. (2001). Remarks from David Satcher, M.D., Ph.D., Assistant Secretary for Health and Surgeon General. *Nutr Rev, 59*(3 Pt 2), S7-9.

U.S. Department of Health and Human Services. (2008). Physical activity guidelines advisory committee report, 2009. Retrieved from www.health.gov/PAGuidelines/Report/Default.aspx

Vos, M. B., & Welsh, J. (2010). Childhood obesity: Update on predisposing factors and prevention strategies. *Curr Gastroenterol Rep, 12*(4), 280-287.

Wang, Y., Beydoun, M.A., Liang, L., Caballero, B., & Kumanyika, S.K. (2008). Will all Americans become overweight or obese? Estimating the progression and cost of the U.S. obesity epidemic. *Obesity (Silver Spring), 16*(10), 2323-2330.

Whitaker, R.C., Wright, J.A., Pepe, M.S., Seidel, K.D., & Dietz, W.H. (1997). Predicting obesity in young adulthood from childhood and parental obesity. *N Engl J Med, 337*(13), 869-873.

World Health Organization. (2003). *Obesity and overweight.* Retrieved from www.who.int/dietphysicalactivity/publications/facts/obesity/en/

World Health Organization. (2006). Global database on body mass index. Retrieved from http://apps.who.int/bmi/index.jsp

World Health Organization. (2010). Global recommendations on physical activity for health. New York: WHO Press.

Zajacova, A. (2008). *Shape of the BMI–mortality association by cause of death using generalized additive models: NHIS 1986-2002. Population Studies Center research report no. 08-639.* Ann Arbor, MI: University of Michigan, Institute for Social Research.

Chapter 3

Adams, G.M. (2002). *Exercise Physiology Laboratory Manual* (4th ed.). New York: McGraw Hill.

Barlow, S.E., & Dietz, W.H. (1998). Obesity evaluation and treatment: Expert committee recommendations. The Maternal and Child Health Bureau Health Resources and Services Administration and the Department of Health and Human Services. *Pediatrics, 102*(3), E29.

Baumgartner, A.K., Zettl, A., Chott, A., Ott, G., Muller-Hermelink, H. K., & Starostik, P. (2003). High frequency of genetic aberrations in enteropathy-type T-cell lymphoma. *Lab Invest, 83*(10), 1509-1516.

Brozek, J., Grande, F., Anderson, J.T., & Keys, A. (1963). Densitometric analysis of body composition: Revision of some quantitative assumptions. *Ann N Y Acad Sci, 110,* 113-140.

Centers for Disease Control and Prevention. (2007a). CDC growth charts: Percentile data files with LMS values. Retrieved from www.cdc.gov/growthcharts/percentile_data_files.htm

Centers for Disease Control and Prevention. (2007b). Healthy weight: It's not a diet, it's a lifestyle! About BMI for adults. Retrieved from www.cdc.gov/healthyweight/assessing/bmi/adult_bmi/index.html

Centers for Disease Control and Prevention. (2007c). Healthy weight: It's not a diet, it's a lifestyle! About BMI for children and teens. Retrieved from www.cdc.gov/healthyweight/assessing/bmi/childrens_bmi/about_childrens_bmi.html

Executive summary of the clinical guidelines on the identification, evaluation, and treatment of overweight and obesity in adults. (1998). *Arch Intern Med, 158*(17), 1855-1867.

Executive summary of the third report of the national cholesterol education program (NCEP) expert panel on detection, evaluation, and treatment of high blood cholesterol in adults (Adult Treatment Panel III). (2001). *JAMA, 285*(19), 2486-2497.

Gallagher, D., Visser, M., Sepulveda, D., Pierson, R.N., Harris, T., & Heymsfield, S.B. (1996). How useful is body mass index for comparison of body fatness across age, sex, and ethnic groups? *Am J Epidemiol, 143*(3), 228-239.

Heyward, V.H., & Wagner, D.R. (2004). *Applied body composition assessment* (2nd ed.). Champaign, IL: Human Kinetics.

Houtkooper, L.B., Lohman, T.G., Going, S.B., & Howell, W.H. (1996). Why bioelectrical imped-ance analysis should be used for estimating adiposity. *Am J Clin Nutr, 64*(3 Suppl), 436S-448S.

Jackson, A.S., Ellis, K.J., McFarlin, B.K., Sailors, M.H., & Bray, M.S. (2009). Body mass index bias in defining obesity of diverse young adults: The Training Intervention and Genetics of Exercise Response (TIGER) study. *British Journal of Nutrition, 102*(7), 1084-1090.

Jackson, A.S., & Pollock, M.L. (1978). Generalized equations for predicting body density of men. *Br J Nutr, 40*(3), 497-504.

Jackson, A.S., Pollock, M.L., & Ward, A. (1980). Generalized equations for predicting body density of women. *Med Sci Sports Exerc, 12*(3), 175-181.

Kaminsky, L.A. (Ed.). (2006). *ACSM's resource manual for guidelines for exercise testing and prescription* (5th ed.). Baltimore: Lippincott Williams and Wilkins.

Nash, H.L. (1985). Body fat measurement: Weighing the pros and cons of electrical impedance. *The Physician and Sports Medicine, 13*(11), 124-128.

Okasora, K., Takaya, R., Tokuda, M., Fukunaga, Y., Oguni, T., Tanaka, H., Konishi, K., & Tamai, H. (1999). Comparison of bioelectrical impedance analysis and dual energy X-ray absorptiometry for assessment of body composition in children. *Pediatr Int, 41*(2), 121-125.

Onishi, N. (2008). Japan, seeking trim waists, measures millions. *New York Times.* Retrieved from www.nytimes.com/2008/06/13/world/asia/13fat.html?_r=2&pagewanted=1

Rexrode, K.M., Carey, V.J., Hennekens, C.H., Walters, E.E., Colditz, G.A., Stampfer, M.J., Willett, W.C., & Manson, J.E. (1998). Abdominal adiposity and coronary heart disease in women. *JAMA, 280*(21), 1843-1848.

Schutte, J.E., Townsend, E.J., Hugg, J., Shoup, R.F., Malina, R.M., & Blomqvist, C.G. (1984). Density of lean body mass is greater in blacks than in whites. *J Appl Physiol, 56*(6), 1647-1649.

Siri, W.E. (1961). Body composition from fluid space and density. In J. Brozek & A. Hanschel (Eds.), *Techniques for measuring body composition* (pp. 223-244). Washington, DC: National Academy of Science.

Slaughter, M.H., Lohman, T.G., Boileau, R.A., Horswill, C.A., Stillman, R.J., Van Loan, M.D., Bemben, D.A. (1988). Skinfold equations for estimation of body fatness in children and youth. *Hum Biol, 60*(5), 709-723.

Tyrrell, V.J., Richards, G., Hofman, P., Gillies, G.F., Robinson, E., & Cutfield, W.S. (2001).

Foot-to-foot bioelectrical impedance analysis: A valuable tool for the measurement of body composition in children. *Int J Obes Relat Metab Disord, 25*(2), 273-278.

Wagner, D.R., & Heyward, V.H. (2000). Measures of body composition in blacks and whites: A comparative review. *Am J Clin Nutr, 71*(6), 1392-1402.

Whaley, M.H. (Ed.). (2006). *ACSM's Guidelines for Exercise Testing and Prescription* (7th ed.). Baltimore: Lippincott Williams and Wilkins.

Chapter 4

Boarnet, M.G., Day, K., Alfonzo, M., Forsyth, A., & Oakes, M. (2006). The Irvine-Minnesota inventory to measure built environments: Reliability tests. *Am J Prev Med, 30*(2), 153-159.

Brownson, R.C., Hoehner, C.M., Brennan, L.K., Cook, R.A., Elliott, M.B., & McMullen, K.M. (2004). Reliability of two instruments for auditing the environment for physical activity. *Journal of physical activity and health, 1*(3), 191-208.

Brownson, R.C., Hoehner, C.M., Day, K., Forsyth, A., & Sallis, J.F. (2009). Measuring the built environment for physical activity: state of the science. *Am J Prev Med, 36*(4 Suppl), S99-123 e112.

Casagrande, S.S., Whitt-Glover, M.C., Lancaster, K.J., Odoms-Young, A.M., & Gary, T.L. (2009). Built environment and health behaviors among African Americans: A systematic review. *Am J Prev Med, 36*(2), 174-181.

Centers for Disease Control and Prevention. (June 2008). Prevention research centers: Mini-grants may maximize health in South Carolina. Retrieved from www.cdc.gov/prc/stories-prevention-research/stories/mini-grants-may-maximize-health.htm

Centers for Disease Control and Prevention. (2007). *Behavioral Risk Factor Surveillance System Survey Data.* Atlanta: U.S. Department of Health and Human Services, Centers for Disease Control and Prevention.

Cerin, E., Saelens, B.E., Sallis, J.F., & Frank, L.D. (2006). Neighborhood Environment Walkability Scale: validity and development of a short form. *Med Sci Sports Exerc, 38*(9), 1682-1691.

Clifton, K.J., Livi Smith, A., & Rodriguez, D. (2007). The Development and Testing of an Audit for the Pedestrian Environment. *Landscape and Urban Planning, 80*(1-2), 95-110.

Duncan, M.J., Spence, J.C., & Mummery, W.K. (2005). Perceived environment and physical activity: a meta-analysis of selected environ-

mental characteristics. *Int J Behav Nutr Phys Act, 2,* 11.

Dunton, G.F., Kaplan, J., Wolch, J., Jerrett, M., & Reynolds, K.D. (2009). Physical environmental correlates of childhood obesity: A systematic review. *Obes Rev, 10*(4), 393-402.

Dwyer, J.J., Allison, K.R., Goldenberg, E.R., Fein, A.J., Yoshida, K.K., & Boutilier, M.A. (2006). Adolescent girls' perceived barriers to participation in physical activity. *Adolescence, 41*(161), 75-89.

ESRI. (2010). What is GIS? Retrieved from www.gis.com/content/what-gis

Feng, J., Glass, T.A., Curriero, F.C., Stewart, W.F., & Schwartz, B.S. (2010). The built environment and obesity: A systematic review of the epidemiologic evidence. *Health Place, 16*(2), 175-190.

Flegal, K.M., Carroll, M.D., Ogden, C.L., & Curtin, L.R. (2010). Prevalence and trends in obesity among US adults, 1999-2008. *JAMA, 303*(3), 235-241.

Frank, L.D., Andresen, M.A., & Schmid, T.L. (2004). Obesity relationships with community design, physical activity, and time spent in cars. *American Journal of Preventive Medicine, 27*(2), 87-96.

Frank, L.D., Engelke, P.O., & Schmidt, T.L. (2003). *Health and community design: The impact of the built environment on physical activity.* Washington, DC: Island Press.

Frank, L.D., Schmid, T.L., Sallis, J.F., Chapman, J., & Saelens, B.E. (2005). Linking objectively measured physical activity with objectively measured urban form: Findings from SMART-RAQ. *American Journal of Preventive Medicine, 28*(2 Suppl 2), 117-125.

Frumkin, H., Frank, L., & Jackson, R. (2004). *Urban sprawl and public health: Designing, planning, and building for healthy communities.* Washington, DC: Island Press.

Gibson, C. (1998). *Population of the 100 largest cities and other urban places in the United States: 1790-1990.* Retrieved from www.census.gov/population/www/documentation/twps0027/twps0027.html#citypop

Gomez, J.E., Johnson, B.A., Selva, M., & Sallis, J.F. (2004). Violent crime and outdoor physical activity among inner-city youth. *Prev Med, 39*(5), 876-881.

Handy, S.L., Boarnet, M.G., Ewing, R., & Killingsworth, R.E. (2002). How the built environment affects physical activity: views from urban planning. *Am J Prev Med, 23*(2 Suppl), 64-73

Heinrich, K.M., Lee, R.E., Regan, G.R., Reese-Smith, J.Y., Howard, H.H., Haddock, C.K.,

Poston, W.S., Poston, W.S., & Ahluwalia, J.S. (2008). How does the built environment relate to body mass index and obesity prevalence among public housing residents? *Am J Health Promot, 22*(3), 187-194.

Heinrich, K.M., Lee, R.E., Suminski, R.R., Regan, G.R., Reese-Smith, J.Y., Howard, H.H., Haddock, C.K. (2007). Associations between the built environment and physical activity in public housing residents. *Int J Behav Nutr Phys Act, 4*, 56.

Jago, R., Baranowski, T., Baranowski, J.C., Thompson, D., & Greaves, K.A. (2005). BMI from 3-6 y of age is predicted by TV viewing and physical activity, not diet. *Int J Obes (Lond), 29*(6), 557-564.

Lavizzo-Mourey, R. (2008). Robert Wood Johnson Foundation 2008 annual report: President's message. Retrieved from www.rwjf.org/files/publications/annual/2008/presidents-message-1.html

Lee, R.E., Liao, Y., & McAlexander, K. (2009). *Associations between neighborhood factors and physical activity in African American public housing residents.* Paper presented at the Urban Affairs Association 2009 Annual Meeting: Contesting and Sustaining the City: Neighborhood, Region, or World. Chicago, IL.

Lumeng, J.C., Appugliese, D., Cabral, H.J., Bradley, R.H., & Zuckerman, B. (2006). Neighborhood safety and overweight status in children. *Arch Pediatr Adolesc Med, 160*(1), 25-31.

McKinnon, R.A., Reedy, J., Morrissette, M.A., Lytle, L.A., & Yaroch, A.L. (2009). Measures of the food environment: A compilation of the literature, 1990-2007. *Am J Prev Med, 36*(4 Suppl), S124-133.

McMillan, T.E., Cubbin, C., Parmenter, B., Medina, A.V., & Lee, R.E. (2010). Neighborhood sampling: how many streets must an auditor walk? *Int J Behav Nutr Phys Act, 7*, 20.

Molnar, B.E., Gortmaker, S.L., Bull, F.C., & Buka, S.L. (2004). Unsafe to play? Neighborhood disorder and lack of safety predict reduced physical activity among urban children and adolescents. *Am J Health Promot, 18*(5), 378-386.

Morland, K., Wing, S., & Diez Roux, A. (2002). The contextual effect of the local food environment on residents' diets: The atherosclerosis risk in communities study. *Am J Public Health, 92*(11), 1761-1767.

Morland, K., Wing, S., Diez Roux, A., & Poole, C. (2002). Neighborhood characteristics associated with the location of food stores and food service places. *Am J Prev Med, 22*(1), 23-29.

Mota, J., Almeida, M., Santos, P., & Ribeiro, J.C. (2005). Perceived neighborhood environments and physical activity in adolescents. *Prev Med, 41*(5-6), 834-836.

National Complete Streets Coalition. (n.d.). Early Successes. Retrieved from www.completestreets.org

Office of the Governor (2008). Governor Schwarzenegger signs sweeping legislation to reduce greenhouse gas emissions through land-use. Retrieved from http://gov.ca.gov/press-release/10697

Ogden, C.L., Carroll, M.D., Curtin, L.R., Lamb, M.M., & Flegal, K.M. (2010). Prevalence of high body mass index in U.S. children and adolescents, 2007-2008. *JAMA, 303*(3), 242-249.

Owen, N., Humpel, N., Leslie, E., Bauman, A., & Sallis, J.F. (2004). Understanding environmental influences on walking; Review and research agenda. *Am J Prev Med, 27*(1), 67-76.

Papas, M.A., Alberg, A.J., Ewing, R., Helzlsouer, K.J., Gary, T.L., & Klassen, A.C. (2007). The built environment and obesity. *Epidemiol Rev, 29*, 129-143.

Pikora, T.J., Bull, F.C., Jamrozik, K., Knuiman, M., Giles-Corti, B., & Donovan, R.J. (2002). Developing a reliable audit instrument to measure the physical environment for physical activity. *Am J Prev Med, 23*(3), 187-194.

Reed, J.A., Wilson, D.K., Ainsworth, B.E., Bowles, H., & Mixon, G. (2006). Perceptions of neighborhood sidewalks on walking and physical activity in southeastern community in the U.S. *Journal of Physical Activity and Health, 3*(2), 243-253.

S. 584: Complete Streets Act of 2009. (2010, February 6). Retrieved from www.govtrack.us/congress/bill.xpd?bill=s111-584

Saelens, B.E., Sallis, J.F., Black, J.B., & Chen, D. (2003). Neighborhood-based differences in physical activity: An environment scale evaluation. *Am J Public Health, 93*(9), 1552-1558.

Sallis, J.F., & Glanz, K. (2006). The role of built environments in physical activity, eating, and obesity in childhood. *Future Child, 16*(1), 89-108.

Sallis, J.F., Saelens, B.E., Frank, L.D., Conway, T.L., Slymen, D.J., Cain, K.L., Chapman, J.E., & Kerr, J. (2009). Neighborhood built environment and income: Examining multiple health outcomes. *Soc Sci Med, 68*(7), 1285-1293.

Sampson, R.J., & Raudenbush, S.W. (2004). Seeing disorder: Neighborhood stigma and the social construction of "broken windows." *Social Psychology Quarterly, 67*(4), 319-342.

Sooman, A., Macintyre, S., & Anderson, A. (1993). Scotland's health: A more difficult challenge for some? The price and availability of healthy foods in socially contrasting localities in the west of Scotland. *Health Bull (Edinb), 51*(5), 276-284.

Strategic Alliance Newsletter (2008, October). Retrieved from www.preventioninstitute.org/sa/103108sanewsletterfull.html#ab31

Troiano, R.P., Berrigan, D., Dodd, K.W., Masse, L.C., Tilert, T., & McDowell, M. (2008). Physical activity in the United States measured by accelerometer. *Med Sci Sports Exerc, 40*(1), 181-188.

Wendel-Vos, W., Droomers, M., Kremers, S., Brug, J., & van Lenthe, F. (2007). Potential environmental determinants of physical activity in adults: A systematic review. *Obes Rev, 8*(5), 425-440.

Chapter 5

Allison, K.R., Dwyer, J.J., Goldenberg, E., Fein, A., Yoshida, K.K., & Boutilier, M. (2005). Male adolescents' reasons for participating in physical activity, barriers to participation, and suggestions for increasing participation. *Adolescence, 40*(157), 155-170.

Bedimo-Rung, A.L., Mowen, A.J., & Cohen, D.A. (2005). The significance of parks to physical activity and public health: A conceptual model. *Am J Prev Med, 28*(2 Suppl 2), 159-168.

Brownson, R.C., Housemann, R.A., Brown, D.R., Jackson-Thompson, J., King, A.C., Malone, B. R., Sallis, J.F. (2000). Promoting physical activity in rural communities: Walking trail access, use, and effects. *Am J Prev Med, 18*(3), 235-241.

Centers for Disease Control and Prevention. (2001). Physical activity trends—United States 1990-1998. *Morb Mortal Wkly Rep, 50*(9), 166-169.

Centers for Disease Control and Prevention. (2007a). CDC growth charts: Percentile data files with LMS values. Retrieved from www.cdc.gov/growthcharts/percentile_data_files.htm

Centers for Disease Control and Prevention. (2007b). Healthy weight: It's not a diet, it's a lifestyle! About BMI for adults. Retrieved from www.cdc.gov/healthyweight/assessing/bmi/adult_bmi/index.html

Cohen, D.A., Ashwood, J.S., Scott, M.M., Overton, A., Evenson, K.R., Staten, L. K., Porter, D., McKenzie, T.L., & Catellier, D. (2006). Public parks and physical activity among adolescent girls. *Pediatrics, 118*(5), e1381-1389.

Cohen, J.E., Planinac, L.C., O'Connor, S.C., Lavack, A.M., Robinson, D.J., & Thompson, F.E. (2008). Keeping the point-of-sale environment at the forefront. *Am J Public Health, 98*(1), 5-6; author reply 6-7.

Cradock, A.L., Kawachi, I., Colditz, G.A., Hannon, C., Melly, S.J., Wiecha, J.L., Gortmaker, S.L. (2005). Playground safety and access in Boston neighborhoods. *Am J Prev Med, 28*(4), 357-363.

Crompton, J.L. (2005). The impact of parks on property values: Empirical evidence from the past two decades in the United States. *Managing Leisure, 10*, 203-218.

Dwyer, J.J., Allison, K.R., Goldenberg, E.R., Fein, A.J., Yoshida, K.K., & Boutilier, M.A. (2006). Adolescent girls' perceived barriers to participation in physical activity. *Adolescence, 41*(161), 75-89.

Eberhardt, M.S., & Pamuk, E.R. (2004). The importance of place of residence: Examining health in rural and nonrural areas. *Am J Public Health, 94*(10), 1682-1686.

Estabrooks, P.A., Lee, R.E., & Gyurcsik, N.C. (2003). Resources for physical activity participation: Does availability and accessibility differ by neighborhood socioeconomic status? *Ann Behav Med, 25*(2), 100-104.

Gobster, P.H., & Dickhut, K.E. (1995). Exploring interspace: Open space opportunities in dense urban areas. In C. K. M. Barrett (Ed.), *Urban Ecosystems: Proceedings of the 7th National Urban Forestry Conference* (pp. 70-73). New York, NY: Washington DC: American Forests.

Ham, S.A., & Epping, J. (2006). Dog walking and physical activity in the United States. *Prev Chronic Dis, 3*(2), A47.

Heinrich, K.M., Lee, R.E., Regan, G.R., Reese-Smith, J.Y., Howard, H.H., Haddock, C.K., Poston, C.S., & Ahluwalia, J.S. (2008). How does the built environment relate to body mass index and obesity prevalence among public housing residents? *Am J Health Promot, 22*(3), 187-194.

Jilcott, S.B., Evenson, K.R., Laraia, B.A., & Ammerman, A.S. (2007). Association between physical activity and proximity to physical activity resources among low-income, midlife women. *Prev Chronic Dis, 4*(1), A04.

Johnson-Down, L., O'Loughlin, J., Koski, K.G., & Gray-Donald, K. (1997). High prevalence of obesity in low income and multiethnic schoolchildren: A diet and physical activity assessment. *J Nutr, 127*(12), 2310-2315.

Kamphuis, C.B., van Lenthe, F.J., Giskes, K., Huisman, M., Brug, J., & Mackenbach, J.P.

(2009). Socioeconomic differences in lack of recreational walking among older adults: The role of neighbourhood and individual factors. *Int J Behav Nutr Phys Act, 6,* 1.

King, A.C., Castro, C., Wilcox, S., Eyler, A.A., Sallis, J.F., & Brownson, R.C. (2000). Personal and environmental factors associated with physical inactivity among different racial-ethnic groups of U.S. middle-aged and older-aged women. *Health Psychol, 19*(4), 354-364.

Lee, R.E., Booth, K.M., Reese-Smith, J.Y., Regan, G., & Howard, H.H. (2005). The Physical Activity Resource Assessment (PARA) instrument: Evaluating features, amenities and incivilities of physical activity resources in urban neighborhoods. *Int J Behav Nutr Phys Act, 2,* 13.

Lee, R.E., Cubbin, C., & Winkleby, M. (2007). Contribution of neighbourhood socioeconomic status and physical activity resources to physical activity among women. *J Epidemiol Community Health, 61*(10), 882-890.

Martin, S.L., Kirkner, G.J., Mayo, K., Matthews, C.E., Durstine, J.L., & Hebert, J.R. (2005). Urban, rural, and regional variations in physical activity. *J Rural Health, 21*(3), 239-244.

McAlexander, K.M., Banda, J.A., McAlexander, J.W., & Lee, R.E. (2009). Physical activity resource attributes and obesity in low-income African Americans. *J Urban Health, 86*(5), 696-707.

Molnar, B.E., Gortmaker, S.L., Bull, F.C., & Buka, S.L. (2004). Unsafe to play? Neighborhood disorder and lack of safety predict reduced physical activity among urban children and adolescents. *Am J Health Promot, 18*(5), 378-386.

Mota, J., Almeida, M., Santos, P., & Ribeiro, J.C. (2005). Perceived neighborhood environments and physical activity in adolescents. *Prev Med, 41*(5-6), 834-836.

Norman, G.J., Nutter, S.K., Ryan, S., Sallis, J.F., Calfras, K.J., & Partrick, K. (2006). Community design and access to recreational facilities as correlates of adolescent physical activity and body-mass index. *Journal of Physical Activity and Health, 3*(1), S118-128.

Office of the Governor (2008). Governor holds press conference to highlight AB 31 and AB 2494 bill signings. Retrieved from http://gov.ca.gov/speech/10733

Owen, N., Humpel, N., Leslie, E., Bauman, A., & Sallis, J.F. (2004). Understanding environmental influences on walking: Review and research agenda. *Am J Prev Med, 27*(1), 67-76.

Parks, S.E., Housemann, R.A., & Brownson, R.C. (2003). Differential correlates of physical activity in urban and rural adults of various socioeconomic backgrounds in the United States. *J Epidemiol Community Health, 57*(1), 29-35.

Powell, L.M., Slater, S., Chaloupka, F.J., & Harper, D. (2006). Availability of physical activity-related facilities and neighborhood demographic and socioeconomic characteristics: A national study. *Am J Public Health, 96*(9), 1676-1680.

Rails-to-Trails Conservancy. (2007). About Rails-to-Trails Conservancy. Retrieved from www.railstotrails.org/index.html

Reed, J.A., & Phillips, D.A. (2005). Relationships between physical activity and the proximity of exercise facilities and home exercise equipment used by undergraduate university students. *J Am Coll Health, 53*(6), 285-290.

Reis, J.P., Bowles, H.R., Ainsworth, B.E., Dubose, K.D., Smith, S., & Laditka, J.N. (2004). Non-occupational physical activity by degree of urbanization and U.S. geographic region. *Med Sci Sports Exerc, 36*(12), 2093-2098.

Saelens, B.E., Frank, L.D., Auffrey, C., Whitaker, R.C., Burdette, H.L., & Colabianchi, N. (2006). Measuring physical environments of parks and playgrounds: EAPRS intrument development and inter-rater reliability. *Journal of Physical Activity & Health, 3*(Suppl 1), S190-S207.

Sallis, J.F., Johnson, M.F., Calfas, K.J., Caparosa, S., & Nichols, J.F. (1997). Assessing perceived physical environmental variables that may influence physical activity. *Res Q Exerc Sport, 68*(4), 345-351.

Sallis, J.F., Patterson, T.L., Buono, M.J., & Nader, P.R. (1988). Relation of cardiovascular fitness and physical activity to cardiovascular disease risk factors in children and adults. *Am J Epidemiol, 127*(5), 933-941.

Sampson, R.J., & Raudenbush, S.W. (2004). Seeing disorder: Neighborhood stigma and the social construction of "broken windows." *Social Psychology Quarterly, 67*(4), 319-342.

San Francisco Bicycle Coalition. (2009). Maps and reference: Tips for the two-wheeled traveler. Retrieved from www.sfbike.org/?maps

Shores, K.A., & West, S.T. (2008). The relationship between built park environments and physical activity in four park locations. *J Public Health Manag Pract, 14*(3), e9-16.

Shores, K.A., & West, S.T. (2010). Rural and urban park visits and park-based physical activity. *Prev Med, 50* (Suppl 1), S13-17.

The Tony Hawk Foundation. (2010). Community impact. Retrieved from www.tonyhawkfoundation.org/about

Troped, P.J., Cromley, E.K., Fragala, M.S., Melly, S J., BHasbrouch, H.H., Gortmarker, S.L., & Brownson, R.C. (2006). Development and reliability and validity testing of an audit tool for train/path characteristics: The path environment audit tool (PEAT). *Journal of Physical Activity & Health, 3*(Suppl 1), S158-S175.

Trost, S.G., Pate, R.R., Ward, D.S., Saunders, R., & Riner, W. (1999). Correlates of objectively measured physical activity in preadolescent youth. *Am J Prev Med, 17*(2), 120-126.

The Trust for Public Land. (2010). Conserving Land for People. Retrieved from www.tpl.org

World Health Organization. (2009). Diet and physical activity: A public health priority, 2009. Retrieved from www.who.int/dietphysicalactivity/en

Zlot, A.I., & Schmid, T.L. (2005). Relationships among community characteristics and walking and bicycling for transportation or recreation. *Am J Health Promot, 19*(4), 314-317.

Chapter 6

Bassett, D.R., Pucher, J., Buehler, R., Thompson, D.L., & Crouter, S.E. (2008). Walking, cycling, and obesity rates in Europe, North America, and Australia. *J Phys Act Health, 5*(6), 795-814.

Besser, L.M., & Dannenberg, A.L. (2005). Walking to public transit: Steps to help meet physical activity recommendations. *Am J Prev Med, 29*(4), 273-280.

Bureau of Transportation Statistics. (2002). National household travel survey 2001-2002. Bureau of Transportation Statistics. Retrieved from www.bts.gov/programs/national_household_travel_survey

Calories per Hour. (2009). Calculating calories burned: Diet and weight loss tutorial. Retrieved from www.caloriesperhour.com/tutorial_net.php

Carver, A., Salmon, J., Campbell, K., Baur, L., Garnett, S., & Crawford, D. (2005). How do perceptions of local neighborhood relate to adolescents' walking and cycling? *Am J Health Promot, 20*(2), 139-147.

Cerin, E., Conway, T.L., Saelens, B.E., Frank, L.D., & Sallis, J.F. (2009). Cross-validation of the factorial structure of the neighborhood environment walkability scale (NEWS) and its abbreviated form (NEWS-A). *Int J Behav Nutr Phys Act, 6*, 32.

Cervero, R., & Kockelman, K.M. (1997). Travel demand and the 3ds: Destiny, diversity, and design. *Transportation Research-D, 2*, 199-219.

Cooper, A.R., Andersen, L.B., Wedderkopp, N., Page, A.S., & Froberg, K. (2005). Physical activity levels of children who walk, cycle, or are driven to school. *Am J Prev Med, 29*(3), 179-184.

Cooper, A.R., Wedderkopp, N., Wang, H., Andersen, L.B., Froberg, K., & Page, A. S. (2006). Active travel to school and cardiovascular fitness in Danish children and adolescents. *Med Sci Sports Exerc, 38*(10), 1724-1731.

Diet Bites. (2009). Calories Burned Climbing Stairs. Retrieved from www.dietbites.com/Pyramid-Diet/calories-burned-climbing-stairs.html

Egana, M., & Donne, B. (2004). Physiological changes following a 12-week gym-based stair-climbing, elliptical trainer, and treadmill running program in females. *J Sports Med Phys Fitness, 44*(2), 141-146.

Eves, F.F., Masters, R.S., & McManus, A.M. (2008). Effects of point-of-choice stair climbing interventions in Hong Kong. *Hong Kong Med J, 14*(5 Suppl), 36-39.

Eves, F.F., Webb, O.J., & Mutrie, N. (2006). A workplace intervention to promote stair climbing: Greater effects in the overweight. *Obesity (Silver Spring), 14*(12), 2210-2216.

Ewing, R., Schmid, T., Killingsworth, R., Zlot, A., & Raudenbush, S. (2003). Relationship between urban sprawl and physical activity, obesity, and morbidity. *Am J Health Promot, 18*(1), 47-57.

Frank, L.D. (2004). Economic determinants of urban form: Resulting trade-offs between active and sedentary forms of travel. *Am J Prev Med, 27*(3 Suppl), 146-153.

Frank, L.D., Andresen, M.A., & Schmid, T.L. (2004). Obesity relationships with community design, physical activity, and time spent in cars. *Am J Prev Med, 27*(2), 87-96.

Frank, L.D., & Engelke, P. (2000). *How land use and transportation systems impact public health: A literature review of the relationship between physical activity and built form.* Atlanta: Georgia Institute of Technology.

Frank, L.D., Engelke, P.O., & Schmidt, T.L. (2003). *Health and community design: The impact of the built environment on physical activty.* Washington, DC: Island Press.

Handy, S.L. (2002). *Accessibility- vs. motility-enhancing strategies for addressing automobile dependence in the U.S.* Paper presented at the European Conference of Ministers of Transport.

Heaner, M. (2009). Does stair climbing bulk up your legs? Retrieved from http://health.msn.

com/fitness/articlepage.aspx?cp-documentid=100241429

Heelan, K.A., Abbey, B. M., Donnelly, J. E., Mayo, M. S., & Welk, G. J. (2009). Evaluation of a walking school bus for promoting physical activity in youth. *J Phys Act Health, 6*(5), 560-567.

Heelan, K.A., Donnelly, J. E., Jacobsen, D. J., Mayo, M. S., Washburn, R., & Greene, L. (2005). Active commuting to and from school and BMI in elementary school children-preliminary data. *Child Care Health Dev, 31*(3), 341-349.

Hinde, S., & Dixon, J. (2005). Changing the obesogenic environment: Insights from a cultural economy of car reliance. *Transportation Research Part D: Transport and Environment, 10*(1), 31-53.

Jacobson, S.H., & McLay, L.A. (2006). The economic impact of obesity on automobile fuel consumption. *The Engineering Economist, 51*(4), 307-323.

Jessup, J.V., Horne, C., Vishen, R.K., & Wheeler, D. (2003). Effects of exercise on bone density, balance, and self-efficacy in older women. *Biol Res Nurs, 4*(3), 171-180.

Kahn, E.B., Ramsey, L.T., Brownson, R.C., Heath, G.W., Howze, E.H., Powell, K.E., Stone, E.J, Rajab, M.W., & Corso, P. (2002). The effectiveness of interventions to increase physical activity: A systematic review. *Am J Prev Med, 22*(4 Suppl), 73-107.

Kerr, J., Rosenberg, D., Sallis, J.F., Saelens, B.E., Frank, L.D., & Conway, T.L. (2006). Active commuting to school: Associations with environment and parental concerns. *Med Sci Sports Exerc, 38*(4), 787-794.

Kong, A.S., Burks, N., Conklin, C., Roldan, C., Skipper, B., Scott, S., et al. (2010). A pilot walking school bus program to prevent obesity in Hispanic elementary school children: Role of physician involvement with the school community. *Clin Pediatr (Phila) 49*(10), 989-991.

Kong, A.S., Sussman, A.L., Negrete, S., Patterson, N., Mittleman, R., & Hough, R. (2009). Implementation of a walking school bus: Lessons learned. *J Sch Health, 79*(7), 319-325; quiz 333-314.

Leyden, K.M. (2003). Social capital and the built environment: The importance of walkable neighborhoods. *Am J Public Health, 93*(9), 1546-1551.

Lopez-Zetina, J., Lee, H., & Friis, R. (2006). The link between obesity and the built environ-

ment. Evidence from an ecological analysis of obesity and vehicle miles of travel in California. *Health Place, 12*(4), 656-664.

McDonald, N.C. (2007). Active transportation to school: Trends among U.S. schoolchildren, 1969-2001. *Am J Prev Med, 32*(6), 509-516.

McDonald, N.C. (2008). Critical factors for active transportation to school among low-income and minority students: Evidence from the 2001 national household travel survey. *Am J Prev Med, 34*(4), 341-344.

Merom, D., Tudor-Locke, C., Bauman, A., & Rissel, C. (2006). Active commuting to school among NSW primary school children: Implications for public health. *Health Place, 12*(4), 678-687.

Moodie, M., Haby, M., Galvin, L., Swinburn, B., & Carter, R. (2009). Cost-effectiveness of active transport for primary school children: Walking school bus program. *Int J Behav Nutr Phys Act, 6*, 63.

Nomura, T., Yoshimoto, Y., Akezaki, Y., & Sato, A. (2009). Changing behavioral patterns to promote physical activity with motivational signs. *Environ Health Prev Med, 14*(1), 20-25.

Olander, E.K., Eves, F.F., & Puig-Ribera, A. (2008). Promoting stair climbing: Stair-riser banners are better than posters . . . sometimes. *Prev Med, 46*(4), 308-310.

Pescatello, L.S., Murphy, D.M., Anderson, D., Costanzo, D., Dulipsingh, L., & De Souza, M.J. (2002). Daily physical movement and bone mineral density among a mixed racial cohort of women. *Med Sci Sports Exerc, 34*(12), 1966-1970.

Powell, L.M., Slater, S., Chaloupka, F.J., & Harper, D. (2006). Availability of physical activity-related facilities and neighborhood demographic and socioeconomic characteristics: A national study. *Am J Public Health, 96*(9), 1676-1680.

Public Health Agency of Canada. (2002). What Is Active Transportation? Retrieved from www.phac-aspc.gc.ca/pau-uap/fitness/active_trans.htm

Puig-Ribera, A., & Eves, F.F. (2010). Promoting stair climbing in Barcelona: Similarities and differences with interventions in English-speaking populations. *Eur J Public Health, 20*(1), 100-102.

Reed, J.A., Wilson, D.K., Ainsworth, B.E., Bowles, H., & Mixon, G. (2006). Perceptions of neighborhood sidewalks on walking and physical activity in southeastern community in the U.S. *Journal of Physical Activity and Health, 3*(2), 243-253.

Rosenberg, D.E., Sallis, J.F., Conway, T.L., Cain, K.L., & McKenzie, T.L. (2006). Active transportation to school over 2 years in relation to weight status and physical activity. *Obesity (Silver Spring), 14*(10), 1771-1776.

Saelens, B.E., & Handy, S.L. (2008). Built environment correlates of walking: A review. *Med Sci Sports Exerc, 40*(7 Suppl), S550-566.

Sallis, J.F., Bauman, A., & Pratt, M. (1998). Environmental and policy interventions to promote physical activity. *Am J Prev Med, 15*(4), 379-397.

Sallis, J.F., & Glanz, K. (2006). The role of built environments in physical activity, eating, and obesity in childhood. *Future Child, 16*(1), 89-108.

Soler, R.E., Leeks, K.D., Buchanan, L.R., Brownson, R.C., Heath, G.W., & Hopkins, D.H. (2010). Point-of-decision prompts to increase stair use: A systematic review update. *Am J Prev Med, 38*(2 Suppl), S292-300.

Southworth, M. (1997). Walkable suburbs? An evaluation of neotraditional communities at the urban edge. *Journal of the American Planning Association, 63*(1), 28-44.

Texas Department of State Health Services (2007). Behavioral risk factor surveillance system data table. Retrieved from www.dshs. state.tx.us/chs/brfss/query/brfss_form.shtm

Timperio, A., Ball, K., Salmon, J., Roberts, R., Giles-Corti, B., Simmons, D.,Baur, L.A., & Crawford, D. (2006). Personal, family, social, and environmental correlates of active commuting to school. *Am J Prev Med, 30*(1), 45-51.

Timperio, A., Salmon, J., Telford, A., & Crawford, D. (2005). Perceptions of local neighbourhood environments and their relationship to childhood overweight and obesity. *Int J Obes (Lond), 29*(2), 170-175.

Transportation Research Board. (2005). Does the built environment influence physical activity? Examining the evidence. Committee on Physical Activity, Health, Transportation, and Land Use. Washington D.C.: Institute of Medicine of the National Academies.

Transport Canada. (2010). "Wheel 2 Work" in Whitehorse. Retrieved from www.tc.gc.ca/eng/programs/environment-utsp-wheel2work-268.htm

Tranter, P.J. (2010). Speed kills: The complex links between transport, lack of time, and urban health. *J Urban Health, 87*(2), 155-166.

U.S. Census Bureau. (2000). American fact finder. Retrieved from http://factfinder.census.gov/servlet/BasicFactsServlet

U.S. Census Bureau News. (2005). Americans spend more than 100 hours commuting to work each year, Census Bureau reports. Retrieved from www.census.gov/newsroom/releases/archives/american_community_survey_acs/cb05-ac02.html

Webb, O.J., & Eves, F.F. (2005). Promoting stair use: Single versus multiple stair-riser messages. *Am J Public Health, 95*(9), 1543-1544.

Webb, O.J., & Eves, F.F. (2007a). Effects of environmental changes in a stair climbing intervention: Generalization to stair descent. *Am J Health Promot, 22*(1), 38-44.

Webb, O.J., & Eves, F.F. (2007b). Promoting stair climbing: Intervention effects generalize to a subsequent stair ascent. *Am J Health Promot, 22*(2), 114-119.

Wen, L.M., & Rissel, C. (2008). Inverse associations between cycling to work, public transport, and overweight and obesity: Findings from a population based study in Australia. *Prev Med, 46*(1), 29-32.

Yancey, A.K., Kumanyika, S.K., Ponce, N.A., McCarthy, W.J., Fielding, J. E., Leslie, J.P., Akbar, J. (2004). Population-based interventions engaging communities of color in healthy eating and active living: A review. *Prev Chronic Dis, 1*(1), A09.

Zhu, X., & Lee, C. (2009). Correlates of walking to school and implications for public policies: Survey results from parents of elementary school children in Austin, Texas. *J Public Health Policy, 30 Suppl 1*, S177-202.

Chapter 7

Barrett, C. B. (2010). Measuring food insecurity. *Science, 327*(5967), 825-828.

Bhargava, A., Jolliffe, D., & Howard, L.L. (2008). Socio-economic, behavioural and environmental factors predicted body weights and household food insecurity scores in the Early Childhood Longitudinal Study—kindergarten. *British Journal of Nutrition 100*(2), 438-444.

Brooks, N., Regmi, A., & Jerardo, A. (2009). U.S. food import patterns, 1998-2007. Retrieved from www.ers.usda.gov/Publications/FAU/2009/08Aug/FAU125/FAU125.pdf

Brownell, K.D. (2007). Should the government tell you what to eat? *Yale Alumni Magazine.* Retrieved from www.yalealumnimagazine.com/issues/2007_07/forum.html

Dixon, J., Omwega, A.M., Friel, S., Burns, C., Donati, K., & Carlisle, R. (2007). The health equity dimensions of urban food systems. *J Urban Health, 84*(3 Suppl), i118-129.

Drewnowski, A., & Darmon, N. (2005). The economics of obesity: Dietary energy density and energy cost. *Am J Clin Nutr, 82*(1 Suppl), 265S-273S.

Elinder, L.S., & Jansson, M. (2009). Obesogenic environments: Aspects on measurement and indicators. *Public Health Nutr, 12*(3), 307-315.

Food and Agriculture Organization of the United Nations. (2002). World Food Summit: Five Years Later. (2002). Retrieved from www.fao.org/worldfoodsummit/english/index.html

Food and Agriculture Organization of the United Nations. (2010). Food security statistics. Retrieved from www.fao.org/economic/ess/food-security-statistics/en

Food Research and Action Center. (2009). Retrieved from www.frac.org

Food System Economic Partnership. (2006). *Macro-level demands and barriers to the creation of local food systems: A preliminary literature review.* Ann Arbor, MI: University of Michigan.

Fox, M.K., Dodd, A.H., Wilson, A., & Gleason, P.M. (2009). Association between school food environment and practices and body mass index of U.S. public school children. *J Am Diet Assoc, 109*(2 Suppl), S108-117.

Francis, C.A., Lieblein, G., Breland, T.A., Salomansson, L., Geber, U., Sriskandarajah, N., Langer, V. (2008). Transdisciplinary research for a sustainable agriculture and food sector. *Agronomy Journal, 100*(3), 771-776.

Hamilton, W.L., Cook, J.T., Thompson, W.W., Buron, L.F., Frongillo, E.A., Olson, C.M., Wehler, C.A. (1997). *Household food security in the United States in 1995: Summary report of the Food Security Measurement Project.* Alexandria: USDA Food and Consumer Service.

Hawkes, C. (2006). Uneven dietary development: Linking the policies and processes of globalization with the nutrition transition, obesity, and diet-related chronic diseases. *Global Health, 2*(4).

Healthy People 2010. (2009). Retrieved from www.healthypeople.gov/default.htm

International Society for Plant Pathology. (2009). Retrieved from www.isppweb.org

Life Sciences Research Office, Inc. (2009). Retrieved from www.lsro.org

Lilliston, B. (2007). *A fair farm bill for America*, Retrieved from www.agobservatory.org/library.cfm?refid=9762

Linz, P., Lee, M., & Bell, L. (2005). Obesity poverty and participation in food and nutrition assiatance programs. Retrieved from www.fns.usda.gov/oane

McDonald's Corporation. (2009). Hungry for McDonald's Nutrition Information? Retrieved from www.mcdonalds.com/us/en/food/food_quality/nutrition_choices.html

MyPyramid. (2008). Inside the Pyramid: How much is my allowance for oils? Retrieved from www.mypyramid.gov/pyramid/oils_allowance_table.html

National Pork Board. (2008). 2008 annual report. Retrieved from www.pork.org/filelibrary/AnnualReport/2008%20Annual%20Report.pdf

National Pork Board. (2009). 2009 annual report. Retrieved from www.pork.org/filelibrary/AnnualReport/AnnualReport2009.pdf

Nestle, M. (2003). Increasing portion sizes in American diets: More calories, more obesity. *J Am Diet Assoc, 103*(1), 39-40.

Nestle, M., & Jacobson, M.F. (2000). Halting the obesity epidemic: A public health policy approach. *Public Health Rep, 115*(1), 12-24.

Nord, M., Andrews, M., & Carlson, S. (2007). Household food security in the United States, 2007. United States Department of Agriculture Economic Research Service. Retrieved from www.ers.usda.gov/Publications/ERR66/ERR66.pdf

Nord, M., Andrews, M., & Carlson, S. (2009). *Household food security in the United States, 2008.* Washington, DC: USDA Economic Research Services.

Ploeq, M.V., Mancino. l., Lin, B. (2006). Food stamps and obesity: Ironic twist or complex puzzle? *Amber waves: The economics of food, farming, natural resources, and rural America.* Retrieved from www.ers.usda.gov/AmberWaves/February06/Features/feature4.htm

Regmi, A., Gehlhar, M., Wainio, J., Vollrath, T., Johnston, P., & Kathuria, N. (2005). Market access for high-value foods. Retrieved from http://151.121.68.30/publications/aer840/aer840.pdf

Ribar, D.C. (2003). Dynamics of poverty and food sufficiency. *Publications.* Retrieved from www.ers.usda.gov/publications/fanrr36

Schlosser, E. (September, 1998). Fast food nation: The true cost of cost of America's diet. *Rolling Stone Magazine.*

Singh, R.B., Pella, D., Mechirova, V., Kartikey, K., Demeester, F., Tomar, R.S., Beegom, R., Mehta, A.S., Gupta, S.B., De Amit, K., Neki, N.S., Haque,

M., Nayse, J., Singh, S., Thakur, A.S., Rastagi, S.S., Singh, K., & Krishna, A. (2007). Prevalence of obesity, physical inactivity and undernutrition, a triple burden of diseases during transition in a developing economy. The Five City Study Group. *Acta Cardiol, 62*(2), 119-127.

Stevenson, M. (2010). Mexico to ban junk food from schools to fight fat. *Associated Press Archive.*

U.S. Department of Agriculture Center for Nutrition Policy and Promotion. (2009). Retrieved from www.cnpp.usda.gov

U.S. Department of Agriculture Economic Research Service. (2007). Food assistance and nutrition programs: RIDGE project summary. Retireved from www.ers.usda.gov/Briefing/FoodNutritionAssistance/funding/RIDGEprojectSummary.asp?Summary_ID=130

U.S. Department of Agriculture Economic Research Service. (2008). Food security in the United States: Measuring household food security. Retrieved from www.ers.usda.gov/Briefing/FoodSecurity/measurement.htm

U.S. Department of Agriculture Food and Nutrtion Service. (2001). National school lunch program: Foods sold in competition with USDA school meal programs. Retrieved from www.fns.usda.gov/cnd/Lunch/_private/CompetitiveFoods/report_congress.htm

U.S. Department of Agriculture Food and Nutrtion Service. (2009a). Child & adult care food program. Retrieved from www.fns.usda.gov/cnd/care

U.S. Department of Agriculture Food and Nutrtion Service. (2009b). National school lunch program. Retrieved from www.fns.usda.gov/cnd/Lunch/default.htm

U.S. Department of Agriculture Food and Nutrtion Service. (2009c). School breakfast program. Retrieved from www.fns.usda.gov/cnd/Breakfast

U.S. Department of Agriculture Food and Nutrtion Service. (2009d). Summer food service program. Retrieved from www.summerfood.usda.gov

U.S. Department of Agriculture Food and Nutrtion Service. (2009e). Supplemental food and nutrition assistance program (SNAP), 2009. Retrieved from www.fns.usda.gov/fsp

U.S. Department of Agriculture Food and Nutrtion Service. (2009f). Women, infants, and children. Retrieved from www.fns.usda.gov/wic

U.S. Department of Agiculture Foreign Agricultural Service. (2006). USDA's Export sales reporting system: Early alert system. Retrieved from www.fas.usda.gov/info/factsheets/expsls.asp

U.S. Department of Commerce Industry report: Food Manufacturing NAICS 311. (2008). Retrieved from www.trade.gov/td/ocg/report08_processedfoods.pdf

Wilde, P.E., McNamara, P.E., & Ranney, C.K. (2000). The effect of dietary quality of participation in the Food Stamp and WIC Programs. Washington, DC: Economic Research Service/USDA.

Woorkman, D. (2008). Most valuable U.S. food export is corn: Japan and Mexico leading countries for American corn imports. Retrieved from http://import-export.suite101.com/article.cfm/most_valuable_us_food_export_is_corn#ixzz0SR2xhNBV

Chapter 8

Akhtar, A.Z., Greger, M., Ferdowsian, H., & Frank, E. (2009). Health professionals' roles in animal agriculture, climate change, and human health. *Am J Prev Med, 36*(2), 182-187.

Associated Press. (2006). What's in that french fry? Fat varies by city. *msnbc.com.* Retrieved from www.msnbc.msn.com/id/12287818

Brown, J.L., & Ping, Y. (2003). Consumer perception of risk associated with eating genetically engineered soybeans is less in the presence of a perceived consumer benefit. *J Am Diet Assoc, 103*(2), 208-214.

Capewell, S., & O'Flaherty, M. (2009). Trends in cardiovascular disease: Are we winning the war? *CMAJ, 180*(13), 1285-1286.

Center for Food Safety. (2009). Retrieved from http://truefoodnow.org

Clevidence, B.A. (2008, March). Weighing in on fats. *Agricultural Research, 56*(3), 12.

Committee on Identifying and Assessing Unintended Effects of Genetically Engineered Foods on Human Health, Board on Life Sciences Food and Nutrition Board, Board on Agriculture and Natural Resources, & Institute of Medicine and National Research Council of the National Academies. (2004). *Safety of genetically engineered foods: Approaches to assessing unintended health effects.* Washington, DC: The National Academies Press.

Curtis, K.R., McCluskey, J.J., & Wahl, T.I. (2004). Consumer acceptance of genetically modified food products in the developing world. *The Journal of Agriobiotechnology Management and Economics, 7*(1&2), 70-75.

Danaei, G., Ding, E.L., Mozaffarian, D., Taylor, B., Rehm, J., Murray, C.J., Ezzati, M. (2009). The preventable causes of death in the United States: Comparative risk assessment of dietary, lifestyle, and metabolic risk factors. *PLoS Med, 6*(4), e1000058.

Eckel, R.H., Borra, S., Lichtenstein, A.H., & Yin-Piazza, S.Y. (2007). Understanding the complexity of trans fatty acid reduction in the American diet: American Heart Association Trans Fat Conference 2006: Report of the Trans Fat Conference Planning Group. *Circulation, 115*(16), 2231-2246.

Fernandez-Cornejo, J., & Caswell, M. (2006). The first decade of genetically engineered crops in the United States. USDA Publications. Retrieved from www.ers.usda.gov/publications/eib11/eib11.pdf

Food and Agriculture Organization of the United Nations. (2000). FAO stresses potential of biotechnology but calls for caution. Retrieved from www.fao.org/WAICENT/OIS/PRESS_NE/PRESSENG/2000/pren0017.htm

Food and Agriculture Organization of the United Nations. (2004). The state of food and agriculture 2003-2004. Retrieved from www.fao.org/docrep/006/y5160e/y5160e00.htm

Food Standards Agency. (2003). *Consumer views of GM food.* England: Food Standards Agency.

Gunther, A.L., Karaolis-Danckert, N., Kroke, A., Remer, T., & Buyken, A.E. (2010). Dietary protein intake throughout childhood is associated with the timing of puberty. *J Nutr, 140*(3), 565-571.

Health Canada. (2005). *The regulation of GM food.* Ottawa: Health Canada.

Hu, F.B., Stampfer, M.J., Manson, J.E., Rimm, E., Colditz, G.A., Rosner, B.A., Hennekens, C.H., & Willett, W.C. (1997). Dietary fat intake and the risk of coronary heart disease in women. *N Engl J Med, 337*(21), 1491-1499.

Human Genome Project. (2008). The science behind the human genome project: Basic genetics, genome draft sequence, and post-genome science. Retrieved from www.ornl.gov/sci/techresources/Human_Genome/project/info.shtml

Kagawa, Y. (1978). Impact of westernization on the nutrition of Japanese: Changes in physique, cancer, longevity and centenarians. *Prev Med, 7*(2), 205-217.

MacIlwain, C. (2000). Rules agreed over GM food exports. *Nature, 403*(6769), 473-474.

Manion-Fischer, K. (2009). States consider trans fat bans, menu labeling. Retrieved from www.stateline.org/live/details/story?contentId=383615

Mauger, J.F., Lichtenstein, A.H., Ausman, L.M., Jalbert, S.M., Jauhiainen, M., Ehnholm, C., Lamarche, B. (2003). Effect of different forms of dietary hydrogenated fats on LDL particle size. *Am J Clin Nutr, 78*(3), 370-375.

Johnson, S.R., Strom, S., & Grillo, K. (2007). *Quantification of the impacts on US agriculture of biotechnology-derived crops planted in 2006.* Washington DC: National Center for Food and Agricultural Policy.

Oeschger, M.P., & Silva, C.E. (2007). Genetically modified organisms in the United States: Implementation, concerns, and public perception. *Adv Biochem Eng Biotechnol, 107*, 57-68.

Okie, S. (2007). New York to trans fats: You're out! *N Engl J Med, 356*(20), 2017-2021.

Paez, K.A., Zhao, L., & Hwang, W. (2009). Rising out-of-pocket spending for chronic conditions: A ten-year trend. *Health Aff (Millwood), 28*(1), 15-25.

Peterson, G., Cunningham, S., Deutsch, L., Erickson, J., Quinlan, A., Raez-Luna, E., Tinch, R.,Troell, M., Woodbury, P., & Zens, S. (2000). The risks and benefits of genetically modified crops: A multidisciplinary perspective. *Conservation Ecology, 4*(1), 13.

Pub. L. No. 75-717, 52 Stat. 1040 (codified as amended at 21 U.S.C. §§ 301-392 (1994)) (1938).

Remer, T., Shi, L., Buyken, A.E., Maser-Gluth, C., Hartmann, M.F., & Wudy, S.A. (2010). Prepubertal adrenarchal androgens and animal protein intake independently and differentially influence pubertal timing. *J Clin Endocrinol Metab, 95*(6), 3002-3009.

Reuters Health. (2009). New York restaurants nearly all trans-fat-free. Retrieved from www.reuters.com/article/idUSTRE56J5HQ20090720

Ross, S.M. (2010). Food for thought, part I: Foodborne illness and factory farming. *Holist Nurs Pract, 24*(3), 169-173.

Saenz de Rodriguez, C.A., Bongiovanni, A.M., & Conde de Borrego, L. (1985). An epidemic of precocious development in Puerto Rican children. *J Pediatr, 107*(3), 393-396.

Semma, M. (2002). Trans fatty acids: properties, benefits and risks. *Journal of Health Science, 48*(1), 7-13.

Sharma, H.C., Sharma, K.K., Seetharama, N., & Ortiz, R. (2000). Prospects for using transgenic resistance to insects in crop improvement. *Electronic Journal of Biotechnology, 3*(2).

Todar, K. (2008). Bacterial resistance to antibiotics. Todar's online textbook of bacteriology.

Retrieved from www.textbookofbacteriology.net/resantimicrobial_4.html

United States Department of Agriculture Economic Research Service. (2009). Adoption of genetically engineered crops in the U.S. Retrieved from www.ers.usda.gov/data/biotechcrops

Urban Harvest. (2010). Urban gardens: Growing gardens, enriching lives. Retrieved from www.urbanharvest.org/index.html

U.S. Department of Health and Human Services. (2009). Federal Food, Drug, and Cosmetic Act (FD&C Act). Retrieved from www.fda.gov/RegulatoryInformation/Legislation/FederalFoodDrugandCosmeticActFDCAct/default.htm

Wolfe, N.D., Dunavan, C.P., & Diamond, J. (2007). Origins of major human infectious diseases. *Nature, 447*(7142), 279-283.

World Health Organization. (2009a). 20 questions on genetically modified (GM) foods. Retrieved from www.who.int/foodsafety/publications/biotech/20questions/en

World Health Organization. (2009b). General information about biotechnology (GM foods). Retrieved from www.who.int/foodsafety/biotech/general/en/index.html

Chapter 9

Action for Healthy Kids. (2009). Retrieved from www.actionforhealthykids.org

Bassett, M.T., Dumanovsky, T., Huang, C., Silver, L.D., Young, C., Nonas, C., Matte, T.D., Chideya, S., & Frieden, T.R. (2008). Purchasing behavior and calorie information at fast-food chains in New York City, 2007. *Am J Public Health, 98*(8), 1457-1459.

Borra, S. (2006). Consumer perspectives on food labels. *Am J Clin Nutr, 83*(5), 1235S.

Burton, S., Creyer, E.H., Kees, J., & Huggins, K. (2006). Attacking the obesity epidemic: The potential health benefits of providing nutrition information in restaurants. *Am J Public Health, 96*(9), 1669-1675.

Connell, D.B., Turner, R.R., & Mason, E.F. (1985). Summary of findings of the School Health Education Evaluation: Health promotion effectiveness, implementation, and costs. *J Sch Health, 55*(8), 316-321.

Drewe, S.B. (1998). Competing conceptions of competition: Implications for physical education *European Physical Education Review, 4*(1), 5-20.

Editorial: Infant and adult obesity. (1974). *Lancet, 1*(7845), 17-18.

Eugeni, M.L., Baxter, M., Mama, S.K., & Lee, R.E. (2010). Disconnections of African American public housing residents: Connections to physical activity, dietary habits and obesity. *American Journal of Community Psychology.*

Fitzgerald, N., Damio, G., Segura-Perez, S., & Perez-Escamilla, R. (2008). Nutrition knowledge, food label use, and food intake patterns among Latinas with and without type 2 diabetes. *J Am Diet Assoc, 108*(6), 960-967.

Flegal, K.M. (2005). Epidemiologic aspects of overweight and obesity in the United States. *Physiol Behav, 86*(5), 599-602.

Flegal, K.M., Carroll, M.D., Ogden, C.L., & Johnson, C.L. (2002). Prevalence and trends in obesity among US adults, 1999-2000. *JAMA, 288*(14), 1723-1727.

Harnack, L.J., French, S.A., Oakes, J.M., Story, M.T., Jeffery, R.W., & Rydell, S.A. (2008). Effects of calorie labeling and value size pricing on fast food meal choices: Results from an experimental trial. *Int J Behav Nutr Phys Act, 5*, 63.

Harrison, K., & Marske, A.L. (2005). Nutritional content of foods advertised during the television programs children watch most. *Am J Public Health, 95*(9), 1568-1574.

Healthy People 2010. (2009). Objective 22: Physical activity and fitness. Retrieved from www.healthypeople.gov/document/html/volume2/22physical.htm

Internal Revenue Service. (2009). Publication 502 (2009), medical and dental expenses. Retrieved from www.irs.gov/publications/p502/index.html

Kuczmarski, R.J., Flegal, K.M., Campbell, S.M., & Johnson, C.L. (1994). Increasing prevalence of overweight among US adults. The National Health and Nutrition Examination Surveys, 1960 to 1991. *JAMA, 272*(3), 205-211.

Lando, A.M., & Labiner-Wolfe, J. (2007). Helping consumers make more healthful food choices: Consumer views on modifying food labels and providing point-of-purchase nutrition information at quick-service restaurants. *J Nutr Educ Behav, 39*(3), 157-163.

Levy, A.S., & Fein, S.B. (1998). Consumers' ability to perform tasks using nutrition labels. *Journal of Nutrition Education and Behavior, 30*(4), 210-217.

McDonald's Corporation. (2010). McDonald's USA nutrition facts for popular menu items. Retrieved from http://nutrition.mcdonalds.com/nutritionexchange/nutritionfacts.pdf

McKenzie, J.F., Pinger, R.R., & Kotecki, J.E. (2005). *An introduction to community health* (5th ed.). Sudbury, MA: Jones and Bartlett Publishers.

Misra, A., & Khurana, L. (2008). Obesity and the metabolic syndrome in developing countries. *J Clin Endocrinol Metab, 93*(11 Suppl 1), S9-30.

Musch, J., & Grondin, S. (2001). Unequal competition as an impediment to personal development: A review of the relative age effect in sport. *Developmental Review, 21*(2), 147-167.

National Association for Sports and Physical Education. (2004). *NASPE: National standards for physical education* (2nd ed.) New York: McGraw Higher Education.

Nestle, M., & Jacobson, M.F. (2000). Halting the obesity epidemic: A public health policy approach. *Public Health Rep, 115*(1), 12-24.

O'Dougherty, M., Harnack, L.J., French, S.A., Story, M., Oakes, J.M., & Jeffery, R.W. (2006). Nutrition labeling and value size pricing at fast-food restaurants: A consumer perspective. *Am J Health Promot, 20*(4), 247-250.

Okosun, I.S., Chandra, K.M., Boev, A., Boltri, J.M., Choi, S.T., Parish, D.C., Dever, G.E. (2004). Abdominal adiposity in U.S. adults: prevalence and trends, 1960-2000. *Prev Med, 39*(1), 197-206.

Popkin, B.M. (1994). The nutrition transition in low-income countries: An emerging crisis. *Nutr Rev, 52*(9), 285-298.

Seidell, J.C. (1995). Obesity in Europe: Scaling an epidemic. *Int J Obes Relat Metab Disord, 19*(Suppl 3), S1-4.

Short, D. (2005). When science met the consumer: The role of industry. *Am J Clin Nutr, 82*(1 Suppl), 256S-258S.

Silventoinen, K., Sans, S., Tolonen, H., Monterde, D., Kuulasmaa, K., Kesteloot, H., Tuomilehto, J. (2004). Trends in obesity and energy supply in the WHO MONICA Project. *Int J Obes Relat Metab Disord, 28*(5), 710-718.

Story, M., Kaphingst, K.M., & French, S. (2006). The role of schools in obesity prevention. *Future Child, 16*(1), 109-142.

Teisl, M.F., & Levy, A.S. (1997). Does nutrition labeling lead to healthier eating? *Journal of Food Distribution Research, 3*(28), 19-26.

U.K. National Food Standards Agency. (2010). Eat well, be well. Retrieved from www.eatwell.gov.uk/foodlabels/trafficlights

United States Department of Agriculture. (2009). Dietary guidelines. Retrieved from www.mypyramid.gov/guidelines/index.html

United States Government Accountability Office. (2008). Food stamp program: Options for delivering financial incentives to participants for purchasing targeted foods. Retrieved from www.gao.gov/new.items/d08415.pdf

U.S. Department of Health and Human Services & U.S. Food and Drug Administration. (2009). Food and drugs, Subpart D: Specific requirements for nutrient content claims. Code of Federal Regulations. *2*(101), 100-102,105-144.

U.S. Department of Health and Human Services & U.S. Department of Agriculture. (2010). Report of the Dietary Guidelines Advisory Committee on the Dietary Guidelines for Americans, 2010. Washington, DC: U.S. Government Printing Office, June 2010.

U.S. Food and Drug Administration. (2009a). International organizations and foreign government agencies. Retrieved from www.fda.gov/InternationalPrograms/Agreements/ucm131179.htm#intlorg

U.S. Food and Drug Administration. (2009b). *Labeling & nutrition.* Retrieved from www.fda.gov/Food/LabelingNutrition/default.htm

U.S. National Physical Activity Plan. (2010). Business and Industry. Retrieved from www.physicalactivityplan.org/business_st5.htm

Variyam, J.N. (2008). Do nutrition labels improve dietary outcomes? *Health Econ, 17*(6), 695-708.

Chapter 10

Adams, F., Wiedmer, P., Gorzelniak, K., Engeli, S., Klaus, S., & Boschmann, M. (2002). Age-related changes of Renin-Angiotensin system genes in white adipose tissue of rats. *Horm Metab Res, 34*(11-12), 716-720.

Aldana, S. G. (2001). Financial impact of health promotion programs: A comprehensive review of the literature. *Am J Health Promot, 15*(5), 296-320.

American Council for an Energy Efficient Economy. (2009). Retrieved from www.aceee.org/press/0908vending.htm

American Heart Association (AHA) Position Statement on effective worksite wellness programs. (2009). Retrieved from www.americanheart.org/downloadable/heart/1213386784466Worksite%20Wellness%20Policy%20Position%20Statement%20to%20NPAM%20and%20EPI.pdf

Bell, A.C., Ge, K., & Popkin, B.M. (2002). The road to obesity or the path to prevention: Motorized transportation and obesity in China. *Obes Res, 10*(4), 277-283.

Bergman, P., Grjibovski, A.M., Hagstromer, M., Patterson, E., & Sjostrom, M. (2010). Congestion road tax and physical activity. *Am J Prev Med, 38*(2), 171-177.

Besser, L.M., & Dannenberg, A.L. (2005). Walking to public transit: Steps to help meet physical activity recommendations. *Am J Prev Med, 29*(4), 273-280.

Chapman, L.S. (2005). Meta-evaluation of worksite health promotion economic return studies: 2005 update. *Am J Health Promot, 19*(6), 1-11.

Chung, C. (1999). Do the poor pay more for food? an analysis of grocery store availability and food price disparities. *Journal Of Consumer Affairs, 33*(2), 276-296.

Clark, S.L., Iceland, J., Palumbo, T., Posey, K., & Weismantle, M. (2003). Comparing employment, income, and poverty: census 2000 and the current population survey. Retrieved from www.census.gov/hhes/www/laborfor/final2_b8_nov6.pdf

Coca-Cola Company. (2007). Coca-Cola Company Annual Report. Retrieved from www.thecoca-colacompany.com/investors/annual_review_2007.html

Commute Trip Reduction Tax Credit. (2005). 59th Legislature Session, State of Washington.

Cullen, K.W., Watson, K., & Zakeri, I. (2008). Improvements in middle school student dietary intake after implementation of the Texas Public School Nutrition Policy. *Am J Public Health, 98*(1), 111-117.

DeMaio, P. (2008, November). The bike-sharing phenomenon—the history of bike-sharing. *Carbusters Magazine, 36*, 12.

Department of Agriculture. (2010). Texas Administrative Code, Title 4, Part 1, Chapter 26, Subchapter A Texas Public School Nutrition Policy. Austin, TX: Texas Secretary of State.

Dodson, E.A., Lovegreen, S.L., Elliott, M.B., Haire-Joshu, D., & Brownson, R.C. (2008). Worksite policies and environments supporting physical activity in midwestern communities. *Am J Health Promot, 23*(1), 51-55.

Eat Smart Move More. (2006). Retrieved from www.eatsmartmovemorenc.com

Hayasaki, E. (2002). Schools to end soda sales; L.A. unified: The soft drinks won't be allowed on campuses starting in 2004. *Los Angeles Times.*

Kahn, E.B., Ramsey, L.T., Brownson, R.C., Heath, G.W., Howze, E.H., Powell, K.E., Stone, E.J., Rajab, M.W., & Corso, P. (2002). The effectiveness of interventions to increase physical activity. A systematic review. *Am J Prev Med, 22*(4 Suppl), 73-107.

Katz, D.L., O'Connell, M., Yeh, M.C., Nawaz, H., Njike, V., Anderson, L.M.,Cory, S., & Dietz, W. (2005). Public health strategies for preventing and controlling overweight and obesity in school and worksite settings: A report on recommendations of the Task Force on Community Preventive Services. *MMWR Recomm Rep, 54*(RR-10), 1-12.

Lankford, T., Kruger, J., & Bauer, D. (2009). State legislation to improve employee wellness. *Am J Health Promot, 23*(4), 283-289.

Lee, R.E., & Cubbin, C. (2009). Striding toward social justice: The ecologic milieu of physical activity. *Exerc Sport Sci Rev, 37*(1), 10-17.

Lopez, R.P., & Hynes, H.P. (2006). Obesity, physical activity, and the urban environment: Public health research needs. *Environ Health, 5*, 25.

Marin Community Foundation. (2009). Retrieved from www.marincf.org

Matson-Koffman, D.M., Brownstein, J.N., Neiner, J.A., & Greaney, M.L. (2005). A site-specific literature review of policy and environmental interventions that promote physical activity and nutrition for cardiovascular health: What works? *Am J Health Promot, 19*(3), 167-193.

Mendoza, J.A., Watson, K., & Cullen, K.W. (2010). Change in dietary energy density after implementation of the Texas Public School Nutrition Policy. *J Am Diet Assoc, 110*(3), 434-440.

Moore, L.V., & Diez Roux, A.V. (2006). Associations of neighborhood characteristics with the location and type of food stores. *Am J Public Health, 96*(2), 325-331.

National Complete Streets Coalition. (2007). Complete Streets Act of 2007. Retrieved from www.completestreets.org

Nestle, M., & Jacobson, M.F. (2000). Halting the obesity epidemic: A public health policy approach. *Public Health Rep, 115*(1), 12-24.

Phipps, E., Madison, N., Pomerantz, S.C., & Klein, M.G. (2010). Identifying and assessing interests and concerns of priority populations for work-site programs to promote physical activity. *Health Promot Pract, 11*(1), 71-78.

Ploeq, M.V. (2006). Food stamps and obesity: Ironic twist or complex puzzle? *Amber waves: the economics of food, farming, natural resources, and rural america.* Retrieved from www.ers.usda.gov/AmberWaves/February06/Features/feature4.htm

Pratt, C.A., Lemon, S.C., Fernandez, I.D., Goetzel, R., Beresford, S.A., French, S.A., Stevens,

V.J., Vogt, T.M., & Webber, L.S. (2007). Design characteristics of worksite environmental interventions for obesity prevention. *Obesity (Silver Spring)*, *15*(9), 2171-2180.

Pucher, J., Dill, J., & Handy, S. (2010). Infrastructure, programs, and policies to increase bicycling: An international review. *Prev Med, 50 Suppl 1*, S106-125.

Sooman, A., Macintyre, S., & Anderson, A. (1993). Scotland's health: A more difficult challenge for some? The price and availability of healthy foods in socially contrasting localities in the west of Scotland. *Health Bull (Edinb)*, *51*(5), 276-284.

Spence, J.C., & Lee, R.E. (2003). Toward a comprehensive model of physical activity. *Psychol Sport Exerc, 4*(1), 7-24.

Stallings, V.A., Suitor, C.W., & Taylor, C.L. (Eds.). (2010). *School meals: building blocks for healthy children*. Washington, DC: Institute of Medicine.

Story, M., Kaphingst, K.M., & French, S. (2006). The role of schools in obesity prevention. *Future Child, 16*(1), 109-142.

Taylor, W.C. (2005). Transforming work breaks to promote health. *Am J Prev Med, 29*(5), 461-465.

U.S. Department of Agriculture. (2002). Farm Bill 2002. Retrieved from www.usda.gov/farm bill2002

USDA Food and Nutrition Service. (2004). Child Nutrition Act amd WIC Reauthorization Act of 2004. Retrieved from www.fns.usda.gov/fdd/legislation/ChildNutandWICReauthActof2004.pdf

Wang, M.C., Kim, S., Gonzalez, A.A., MacLeod, K.E., & Winkleby, M.A. (2007). Socioeconomic and food-related physical characteristics of the neighbourhood environment are associated with body mass index. *J Epidemiol Community Health, 61*(6), 491-498.

Weber, J.A., & Becker, N. (2006). Framing the farm bill. *J Am Diet Assoc, 106*(9), 1354, 1356-1357.

Wen, L.M., & Rissel, C. (2008). Inverse associations between cycling to work, public transport, and overweight and obesity: Findings from a population based study in Australia. *Prev Med, 46*(1), 29-32.

Zenk, S.N., Schulz, A.J., Israel, B.A., James, S.A., Bao, S., & Wilson, M.L. (2005). Neighborhood racial composition, neighborhood poverty, and the spatial accessibility of supermarkets in metropolitan Detroit. *Am J Public Health, 95*(4), 660-667.

Chapter 11

Airhihenbuwa, C.O., Kumanyika, S., Agurs, T.D., Lowe, A., Saunders, D., & Morssink, C.B. (1996). Cultural aspects of African American eating patterns. *Ethn Health, 1*(3), 245-260.

Anschutz, D.J., Engels, R.C., Becker, E.S., & van Strien, T. (2008). The bold and the beautiful: Influence of body size of televised media models on body dissatisfaction and actual food intake. *Appetite, 51*(3), 530-537.

Bennett, E.M. (1991). Weight-loss practices of overweight adults. *Am J Clin Nutr, 53*(6 Suppl), 1519S-1521S.

Bindon, J., Dressler, W.W., Gilliland, M.J., & Crews, D.E. (2007). A cross-cultural perspective on obesity and health in three groups of women: The Mississippi Choctaw, American Samoans, and African Americans. *Coll Antropol, 31*(1), 47-54.

Birch, L.L., & Davison, K.K. (2001). Family environmental factors influencing the developing behavioral controls of food intake and childhood overweight. *Pediatr Clin North Am, 48*(4), 893-907.

Bouchard, C. (1997). Genetic determinants of regional fat distribution. *Hum Reprod, 12* (Suppl 1), 1-5.

Bruss, M.B., Morris, J., & Dannison, L. (2003). Prevention of childhood obesity: Sociocultural and familial factors. *J Am Diet Assoc, 103*(8), 1042-1045.

Chen, J.L., & Kennedy, C. (2002). Functioning, parenting style, and Chinese children's weight status. *Journal of Family Nursing, 10*(2), 262-279.

Crossman, A., Anne Sullivan, D., & Benin, M. (2006). The family environment and American adolescents' risk of obesity as young adults. *Soc Sci Med, 63*(9), 2255-2267.

Eatoutzone. (2007). Cuisine of Africa. Retrieved from www.eatoutzone.com/African_Cuisine.htm

Egger, G., & Swinburn, B. (1997). An "ecological" approach to the obesity pandemic. *BMJ, 315*(7106), 477-480.

Epstein, L.H., Valoski, A., Koeske, R., & Wing, R.R. (1986). Family-based behavioral weight control in obese young children. *J Am Diet Assoc, 86*(4), 481-484.

Flegal, K.M., Carroll, M.D., Ogden, C.L., & Johnson, C.L. (2010). Prevalence and trends in obesity among US adults, 1999-2008. *JAMA, 303*(3), 235-241.

Ford, P.B., & Dzewaltowski, D.A. (2008). Disparities in obesity prevalence due to variation in the retail food environment: Three testable hypotheses. *Nutr Rev, 66*(4), 216-228.

Harris, M.B., Walters, L.C., & Waschull, S. (1991). Gender and ethnic differences in obesity related behaviors and attitudes in a college sample. *Journal of Applied Social Psychology, 21*(19), 1545-1566.

Haslam, D.W., & James, W.P. (2005). Obesity. *Lancet, 366*(9492), 1197-1209.

Heinrich, K.M., Lee, R.E., Regan, G.R., Reese-Smith, J.Y., Howard, H.H., Haddock, C.K. Poston, W.S., & Ahluwalia, J.S. (2008). How does the built environment relate to body mass index and obesity prevalence among public housing residents? *Am J Health Promot, 22*(3), 187-194.

Henderson, K.A., & Ainsworth, B.E. (2003). A synthesis of perceptions about physical activity among older African American and American Indian women. *Am J Public Health, 93*(2), 313-317.

Khanam, S., & Costarelli, V. (2008). Attitudes towards health and exercise of overweight women. *J R Soc Promot Health, 128*(1), 26-30.

Kumanyika, S. (1987). Obesity in black women. *Epidemiol Rev, 9*, 31-50.

Kumanyika, S. (1993). Ethnicity and obesity development in children. *Ann N Y Acad Sci, 699*, 81-92.

Kumanyika, S., & Ewart (1990). Theoretical and baseline considerations for diet and weight control of diabetes among blacks. *Diabetes Care, 13*(11), 1154–1162

Kumanyika, S., Morssink, C., & Agurs, T. (1992). Models for dietary and weight change in African-American women: Identifying cultural components. *Ethn Dis, 2*(2), 166-175.

Laskarzewski, P.M., Khoury, P., Morrison, J.A., Kelly, K., Mellies, M.J., & Glueck, C.J. (1983). Familial obesity and leanness. *Int J Obes, 7*(6), 505-527.

Lee, R.E., & Cubbin, C. (2002). Neighborhood context and youth cardiovascular health behaviors. *Am J Public Health, 92*(3), 428-436.

Lee, R.E., Heinrich, K.M., Medina, A.V., Maddock, J.E., Regan, G.R., & Reese-Smith, J.Y. (2009). Healthful food environment in two diverse urban cities: Same same only different? *Environ Health Insights, 4*, 49-60.

Mainous, A.G., 3rd, Diaz, V.A., & Geesey, M.E. (2008). Acculturation and healthy lifestyle among Latinos with diabetes. *Ann Fam Med, 6*(2), 131-137.

Melnyk, M.G., & Weinstein, E. (1994). Preventing obesity in black women by targeting ado-

lescents: a literature review. *J Am Diet Assoc, 94*(5), 536-540.

Merten, M.J., Williams, A.L., & Shriver, L.H. (2009). Breakfast consumption in adolescence and young adulthood: Parental presence, community context, and obesity. *J Am Diet Assoc, 109*(8), 1384-1391.

Neff, L.J., Sargent, R.G., McKeown, R.E., Jackson, K.L., & Valois, R.F. (1997). Black-white differences in body size perceptions and weight management practices among adolescent females. *J Adolesc Health, 20*(6), 459-465.

Nielsen, S.J., & Popkin, B.M. (2003). Patterns and trends in food portion sizes, 1977-1998. *JAMA, 289*(4), 450-453.

Olson, C.M., Bove, C.F., & Miller, E.O. (2007). Growing up poor: Long-term implications for eating patterns and body weight. *Appetite, 49*(1), 198-207.

Perez-Escamilla, R., & Putnik, P. (2007). The role of acculturation in nutrition, lifestyle, and incidence of type 2 diabetes among Latinos. *J Nutr, 137*(4), 860-870.

Pinhey, T.K., Rubenstein, D.H., & Colfax, R.S. (1997). Overweight and happiness: The reflected self-appraisal hypothesis reconsidered: Consequences of obesity. *Social Science Quarterly, 78*(3), 747-755.

Popkin, B.M., & Udry, J.R. (1998). Adolescent obesity increases significantly in second and third generation U.S. immigrants: The national longitudinal study of adolescent health. *J Nutr, 128*(4), 701-706.

Prentice, A.M., & Jebb, S.A. (2003). Fast foods, energy density and obesity: A possible mechanistic link. *Obes Rev, 4*(4), 187-194.

Regan, G., Lee, R.E., Booth, K., & Reese-Smith, J. (2006). Obesogenic influences in public housing: A mixed-method analysis. *Am J Health Promot, 20*(4), 282-290.

Richter, D.L., Wilcox, S., Greaney, M.L., Henderson, K.A., & Ainsworth, B.E. (2002). Environmental, policy, and cultural factors related to physical activity in African American women. *Women Health, 36*(2), 91-109.

Sankofa, J., & Johnson-Taylor, W.L. (2007). News coverage of diet-related health disparities experienced by black americans: A steady diet of misinformation. *J Nutr Educ Behav, 39*(2 Suppl), S41-44.

Savage, J.S., Fisher, J.O., & Birch, L.L. (2007). Parental influence on eating behavior: Conception to adolescence. *J Law Med Ethics, 35*(1), 22-34.

Smith, C., & Richards, R. (2008). Dietary intake, overweight status, and perceptions of food insecurity among homeless Minnesotan youth. *Am J Hum Biol, 20*(5), 550-563.

Spence, J.C., & Lee, R.E. (2003). Toward a comprehensive model of physical activity. *Psychol Sport Exerc, 4*(1), 7-24.

Strauss, R.S., & Knight, J. (1999). Influence of the home environment on the development of obesity in children. *Pediatrics, 103*(6), e85.

Thomas, V.G., & James, M.D. (1988). Body image, dieting tendencies, and sex roles. *Sex Roles, 18*, 523-529.

Treuth, M.S., Butte, N.F., & Sorkin, J.D. (2003). Predictors of body fat gain in nonobese girls with a familial predisposition to obesity. *Am J Clin Nutr, 78*(6), 1212-1218.

Tudor-Locke, C., Henderson, K.A., Wilcox, S., Cooper, R.S., Durstine, J.L., & Ainsworth, B.E. (2003). In their own voices: Definitions and interpretations of physical activity. *Womens Health Issues, 13*(5), 194-199.

U.S. Department of Health and Human Services. (2010). We Can. Retrieved from www.nhlbi.nih.gov/health/public/heart/obesity/wecan/about-wecan/index.htm

U.S. Department of Health and Human Services & Centers for Disease Control and Prevention. (2010). Healthy Families Calendar: 2010 Safe and Healthy Families. Retrieved from www.cdc.gov/family/calendar/families_sp_11x17.pdf

Ventura, A.K., & Birch, L.L. (2008). Does parenting affect children's eating and weight status? *Int J Behav Nutr Phys Act, 5*(15).

Wells, J.C. (2006). The evolution of human fatness and susceptibility to obesity: An ethological approach. *Biol Rev Camb Philos Soc, 81*(2), 183-205.

Wilbur, J., Chandler, P.J., Dancy, B., & Lee, H. (2003). Correlates of physical activity in urban midwestern Latinas. *Am J Prev Med, 25*(3 Suppl 1), 69-76.

Yuasa, K., Sei, M., Takeda, E., Ewis, A.A., Munakata, H., Onishi, C., Nakahori, Y. (2008). Effects of lifestyle habits and eating meals together with the family on the prevalence of obesity among school children in Tokushima, Japan: A cross-sectional questionnaire-based survey. *J Med Invest, 55*(1-2), 71-77.

Chapter 12

Access to healthy foods in low-income neighborhoods: Opportunities for public policy. (2008).

New Haven, CT: Rudd Center for Food Policy & Obesity.

Adler, N.E., Boyce, T., Chesney, M.A., Cohen, S., Folkman, S., Kahn, R.L., Syme, S.L. (1994). Socioeconomic status and health. The challenge of the gradient. *Am Psychol, 49*(1), 15-24.

Anderson, L., Scrimshaw, S., Fullilove, M., and Fielding, J. (2003). "The Community Guide's model for linking the social environment to health," *American Journal of Preventive Medicine, 24*(3S), 12-20.

Andreyeva, T., Puhl, R.M., & Brownell, K.D. (2008). Changes in perceived weight discrimination among Americans, 1995-1996 through 2004-2006. *Obesity (Silver Spring), 16*(5), 1129-1134.

Artazcoz, L., Cortes, I., Escriba-Aguir, V., Cascant, L., & Villegas, R. (2009). Understanding the relationship of long working hours with health status and health-related behaviours. *J Epidemiol Community Health, 63*(7), 521-527.

Bassett, M.T., Dumanovsky, T., Huang, C., Silver, L.D., Young, C., Nonas, C., Matte, T.D., Chideya, S., & Frieden, T.R. (2008). Purchasing behavior and calorie information at fast-food chains in New York City, 2007. *Am J Public Health, 98*(8), 1457-1459.

Blue Cross and Blue Shield of Minnesota Foundation. (n.d.). Determinants and critical pathways charts. Retrieved from www.bcbsmnfoundation.org/objects/Tier_4/mbc2_determinants_charts.pdf

Boushey, H., Fremstad, S., Gragg, R., & Waller, M. (2007). *The mobility agenda: a special initiative of inclusion and the center for economic policy and research, understanding low-wage work in the United States.* Washington, DC: Center for Economic Policy and Research.

Braveman, P., & Gruskin, S. (2003). Defining equity in health. *J Epidemiol Community Health, 57*(4), 254-258.

Braveman, P.A., Cubbin, C., Egerter, S., Chideya, S., Marchi, K.S., Metzler, M., Posner, S. (2005). Socioeconomic status in health research: One size does not fit all. *JAMA, 294*(22), 2879-2888.

Centers for Disease Control and Prevention (2009). *Nutrition, physical activity and obesity state and program examples.* Atlanta, GA: Centers for Disease Control and Prevention.

Cossrow, N.H., Jeffery, R.W., & McGuire, M. T. (2001). Understanding weight stigmatization: A focus group study. *J Nutr Educ, 33*(4), 208-214.

Cubbin, C., Hadden, W. C., & Winkleby, M. A. (2001). Neighborhood context and cardiovas-

cular disease risk factors: The contribution of material deprivation. *Ethn Dis, 11*(4), 687-700.

Cubbin, C., Sundquist, K., Ahlen, H., Johansson, S. E., Winkleby, M. A., & Sundquist, J. (2006). Neighborhood deprivation and cardiovascular disease risk factors: Protective and harmful effects. *Scand J Public Health, 34*(3), 228-237.

Dodson, L., & Bravo, E. (2005). When there is no time or money: work, family, and community lives of low-income families. In Christopher Beem and Jody Heymann (Eds.), *Unfinished work: Building democracy and equality in an era of working families*. New York: The New Press.

Ehrenreich, B. (2001). *Nickel and dimed: On (not) getting by in America*. New York, NY: Metropolitan Books.

Estabrooks, P.A., Lee, R.E., & Gyurcsik, N.C. (2003). Resources for physical activity participation: Does availability and accessibility differ by neighborhood socioeconomic status? *Ann Behav Med, 25*(2), 100-104.

Foster, G.D., Wadden, T.A., Makris, A.P., Davidson, D., Sanderson, R.S., Allison, D.B., Kessler, A. (2003). Primary care physicians' attitudes about obesity and its treatment. *Obes Res, 11*(10), 1168-1177.

Frank, L.D., Andresen, M.A., & Schmid, T.L. (2004). Obesity relationships with community design, physical activity, and time spent in cars. *Am J Prev Med, 27*(2), 87-96.

Gallo, L.C., Penedo, F.J., Espinosa de los Monteros, K., & Arguelles, W. (2009). Resiliency in the face of disadvantage: Do Hispanic cultural characteristics protect health outcomes? *J Pers, 77*(6), 1707-1746.

Health Resources and Services Administration. (2008). Health literacy. Retrieved from www.hrsa.gov/healthliteracy/

Hebl, M.R., & Xu, J. (2001). Weighing the care: Physicians' reactions to the size of a patient. *Int J Obes Relat Metab Disord, 25*(8), 1246-1252.

Heinrich, K.M., Lee, R.E., Regan, G.R., Reese-Smith, J.Y., Howard, H.H., Haddock, C.K., Poston, W.S. (2008). How does the built environment relate to body mass index and obesity prevalence among public housing residents? *Am J Health Promot, 22*(3), 187-194.

Henry, J.P. (1988). Stress, salt and hypertension. *Soc Sci Med, 26*(3), 293-302.

Kennen, E.M., Davis, T.C., Huang, J., Yu, H., Carden, D., Bass, R., Arnold, C. (2005). Tipping the scales: The effect of literacy on obese patients' knowledge and readiness to lose weight. *South Med J, 98*(1), 15-18.

Keyes, C.L. (2009). The Black-White paradox in health: Flourishing in the face of social inequality and discrimination. *J Pers, 77*(6), 1677-1706.

Lee, R.E., Booth, K.M., Reese-Smith, J.Y., Regan, G., & Howard, H.H. (2005). The Physical Activity Resource Assessment (PARA) instrument: Evaluating features, amenities and incivilities of physical activity resources in urban neighborhoods. *Int J Behav Nutr Phys Act, 2*, 13.

Lee, R.E., & Cubbin, C. (2002). Neighborhood context and youth cardiovascular health behaviors. *Am J Public Health, 92*(3), 428-436.

Lee, R.E., & Cubbin, C. (2009). Striding toward social justice: The ecologic milieu of physical activity. *Exerc Sport Sci Rev, 37*(1), 10-17.

Lee, R.E., Greiner, K.A., Hall, S., Born, W., Kimminau, K.S., Allison, A., & Ahluwalia, J.S. (2007). Ecologic correlates of obesity in rural obese adults. *J Am Coll Nutr, 26*(5), 424-433.

Link, B.G., & Phelan, J.C. (2002). McKeown and the idea that social conditions are fundamental causes of disease. *Am J Public Health, 92*(5), 730-732.

Loera, A. (2009). Pantry upgrade, 2009. Retrieved from www.rezoom.com/health/read/5417

Marin Community Foundation. (2009). Retrieved from www.marincf.org

Marin, G., & Marin, B.V. (1991). *Research with Hispanic populations*. Newbury Park: Sage.

Martinez, M.C., & Fischer, F.M. (2009). Stress at work among electric utility workers. *Ind Health, 47*(1), 55-63.

McDonald, N.C. (2007). Active transportation to school: Trends among U.S. schoolchildren, 1969-2001. *Am J Prev Med, 32*(6), 509-516.

Morland, K., & Filomena, S. (2007). Disparities in the availability of fruits and vegetables between racially segregated urban neighbourhoods. *Public Health Nutr, 10*(12), 1481-1489.

Muijs, D., Harris, A., Chapman, C., Stoll, L., & Russ, J. (2004). Improving schools in socioeconomically disadvantaged areas: A review of the research evidence *School Effectiveness and School Improvement 15*(2), 149-175.

Nandi, P.K., & Harris, H. (1999). The social world of female-headed black families: A study of quality of life in a marginalized neighborhood. *International Journal of Comparative Sociology, 40*.

National Network of Libraries of Medicine. (2010). Healthy people 2010. Retrieved from http://nnlm.gov/outreach/consumer/hlthlit.html#A1

NIH Centers for Population Health and Health Disparities. (2009). Retrieved from http://can-

cercontrol.cancer.gov/populationhealthcenters/cphhd/centers.html

Ogden, C.L., Carroll, M.D., Curtin, L.R., McDowell, M.A., Tabak, C.J., & Flegal, K.M. (2006). Prevalence of overweight and obesity in the United States, 1999-2004. *JAMA, 295*(13), 1549-1555.

Popkin, B.M., & Doak, C.M. (1998). The obesity epidemic is a worldwide phenomenon. *Nutr Rev, 56*(4 Pt 1), 106-114.

Prus, S.G. (2007). Age, SES, and health: A population level analysis of health inequalities over the lifecourse. *Sociol Health Illn, 29*(2), 275-296.

Puhl, R., & Brownell, K.D. (2003). Ways of coping with obesity stigma: Review and conceptual analysis. *Eat Behav, 4*(1), 53-78.

Roehling, M., Roehling, P., & Pichler, S. (2007). The relationship between body weight and perceived weight-related employment discrimination: The role of sex and race. *Journal of Vocational Behavior, 71*(2), 300-318.

Rosenberg, D.E., Sallis, J.F., Conway, T.L., Cain, K.L., & McKenzie, T.L. (2006). Active transportation to school over 2 years in relation to weight status and physical activity. *Obesity (Silver Spring), 14*(10), 1771-1776.

U.S. Census Bureau. (2009). Estimates of the Resident Population by Race and Hispanic Origin for the United States and States 2009. Retrieved from www.census.gov/popest/states/asrh/SC-EST2009-04.html

U.S. Department of Education National Center for Education Statistics. (2008). *The Condition of Education 2008.* Washington, DC: U.S. Department of Education National Center for Education Statistics.

U.S. Department of Health and Human Services. (1996). *Physical activity and health: A report of the Surgeon General.* Atlanta: Centers for Disease Control and Prevention.

Wang, Y. (2001). Cross-national comparison of childhood obesity: the epidemic and the relationship between obesity and socioeconomic status. *Int J Epidemiol, 30*(5), 1129-1136.

Williams, D.A., & Collins, C. (1995). US socioeconomic and racial differences in health: Patterns and explanations. *Annu Rev Sociol, 21*, 349-386.

Chapter 13

American Marketing Association. (2009). Resource library dictionary. Retrieved from www.marketingpower.com/_layouts/Dictionary.aspx

Chung, C. (1999). Do the poor pay more for food? An analysis of grocery store availability and food price disparities. *Journal of Consumer Affairs, 33*(2), 276-296.

Cummins, S., & Macintyre, S. (2006). Food environments and obesity: Neighbourhood or nation? *International Journal of Epidemiology, 35*(1), 100-104.

Diez-Roux, A.V., Nieto, F.J., Caulfield, L., Tyroler, H.A., Watson, R.L., & Szklo, M. (1999). Neighbourhood differences in diet: The Atherosclerosis Risk in Communities (ARIC) Study. *Journal Epidemiol Community Health, 53*(1), 55-63.

Drewnowski, A., & Darmon, N. (2005). The economics of obesity: Dietary energy density and energy cost. *Am J Clin Nutr, 82*(1 Suppl), 265S-273S.

Ellaway, A., & Macintyre, S. (1996). Does where you live predict health related behaviours? A case study in Glasgow. *Health Bulletin (Edinb), 54*(6), 443-446.

Jetter, K.M., & Cassady, D.L. (2006). The availability and cost of healthier food alternatives. *Am J Prev Med, 30*(1), 38-44.

Kunkel, D., McKinley, C., & Wright, P. (2009). The impact of industry self-regulation on the nutritional quality of foods advertised on television to children. Retrieved from www.foodpolitics.com/wp-content/uploads/adstudy09_report-1.pdf

Latham, J., & Moffat, T. (2007). Determinants of variation in food cost and availability in two socioeconomically contrasting neighbourhoods of Hamilton, Ontario, Canada. *Health Place, 13*(1), 273-287.

Lee, R.E., & Cubbin, C. (2002). Neighborhood context and youth cardiovascular health behaviors. *Am J Public Health, 92*(3), 428-436.

Meyers Research Center. (1995). Point-of-Purchase Advertising Institute (POPAI) consumer habits buying study. New York, NY: Meyers Research Center.

Mooney, C. (1990). Cost and availability of healthy food choices in a London health district. *J Hum Nutr Diet, 3*(2), 111-120.

Moore, L.V., & Diez Roux, A.V. (2006). Associations of neighborhood characteristics with the location and type of food stores. *Am J Public Health, 96*(2), 325-331.

Poston, W.S., & Foreyt, J.P. (1999). Obesity is an environmental issue. *Atherosclerosis, 146*(2), 201-209.

Sooman, A., Macintyre, S., & Anderson, A. (1993). Scotland's health: A more difficult challenge for some? The price and availability of healthy foods in socially contrasting localities in the west of Scotland. *Health Bull (Edinb), 51*(5), 276-284.

United States Department of Health and Human Services (USDHHS). (2009). Federal Food, Drug, and Cosmetic Act (FD&C Act). Retrieved from www.fda.gov/RegulatoryInformation/ Legislation/FederalFoodDrugandCosmeti-cActFDCAct/default.htm

Wang, M.C., Kim, S., Gonzalez, A.A., MacLeod, K.E., & Winkleby, M.A. (2007). Socioeconomic and food-related physical characteristics of the neighbourhood environment are associated with body mass index. *J Epidemiol Community Health, 61*(6), 491-498.

White, M.J. (1987). *American neighborhoods and residential differentiation.* New York: Russell Sage Foundation.

Who's Minding the Shelves? (2000). *Consumer Reports, 65*(i8), 8.

Zenk, S.N., Schulz, A.J., Israel, B.A., James, S.A., Bao, S., & Wilson, M.L. (2005). Neighborhood racial composition, neighborhood poverty, and the spatial accessibility of supermarkets in metropolitan Detroit. *Am J Public Health, 95*(4), 660-667.

Zhang, Q., & Wang, Y. (2004). Trends in the association between obesity and socioeconomic status in U.S. adults: 1971 to 2000. *Obes Res, 12*(10), 1622-1632.

Chapter 14

Alvy, L.M., & Calvert, S.L. (2008). Food marketing on popular children's web sites: A content analysis. *J Am Diet Assoc, 108*(4), 710-713.

American Dietetic Association. (2006). Position paper update for 2006. *Journal of the American Dietetic Association, 106*(2), 294-295.

Anderson, A.S., Porteous, L.E., Foster, E., Higgins, C., Stead, M., Hetherington, M., Ha, M.A., & Adamson, A.J. (2005). The impact of a school-based nutrition education intervention on dietary intake and cognitive and attitudinal variables relating to fruits and vegetables. *Public Health Nutr, 8*(6), 650-656.

Anschutz, D.J., Engels, R.C., & Van Strien, T. (2009). Side effects of television food commercials on concurrent nonadvertised sweet snack food intakes in young children. *Am J Clin Nutr, 89*(5), 1328-1333.

Bennett, G.G., Wolin, K.Y., Viswanath, K., Askew, S., Puleo, E., & Emmons, K.M. (2006). Television viewing and pedometer-determined physical activity among multiethnic residents of low-income housing. *Am J Public Health, 96*(9), 1681-1685.

Burdette, H.L., & Whitaker, R.C. (2005). A national study of neighborhood safety, outdoor play, television viewing, and obesity in preschool children. *Pediatrics, 116*(3), 657-662.

Bureau of Labor Statistics. (2009). American time use survey summary: 2008 results. Retrieved from www.bls.gov/news.release/atus.nr0.htm

Centers for Disease Control and Prevention. (2009). Eat a variety of fruits and vegetables every day. Retrieved from www.fruitsandveggiesmatter.gov

Children's TV Network. (2009). Retrieved from http://childrenstvnetwork.com

Chou, S.Y., Rashad, I., & Grossman, M. (2008). Fast food restaurant advertising on television and its influence on childhood obesity. [Electronic version]. *Journal of Law and Economics, 51*(4), 599-618.

Connor, S.M. (2006). Food-related advertising on preschool television: building brand recognition in young viewers. *Pediatrics, 118*(4), 1478-1485.

Coon, K.A., Goldberg, J., Rogers, B.L., & Tucker, K.L. (2001). Relationships between use of television during meals and children's food consumption patterns. *Pediatrics, 107*(1), E7.

Dennison, B.A., Erb, T.A., & Jenkins, P.L. (2002). Television viewing and television in bedroom associated with overweight risk among low-income preschool children. *Pediatrics, 109*(6), 1028-1035.

Division of Community Health, Nutrition Training Institute. (2005). Media literacy: An innovative approach for prevention and management of childhood overweight. Jefferson City, MO: State of Missouri Department of Health and Senior Services.

Dixon, H.G., Scully, M.L., Wakefield, M.A., White, V.M., & Crawford, D.A. (2007). The effects of television advertisements for junk food versus nutritious food on children's food attitudes and preferences. *Soc Sci Med, 65*(7), 1311-1323.

Dunstan, D.W., Barr, E.L. M., Healy, G.N., Salmon, J., Shaw, J.E., Balkau, B., Magliano, D.J.,Cameron, A.J., Zimmet, P.Z., & Owen, N. (2010). Television viewing time and mortality: The Australian diabetes, obesity and lifestyle study (AusDiab). *Circulation, 121*(3), 384-391.

Epstein , L.H., Roemmich, J.N., Robinson, J.L., Paluch, R.A., Winiewicz, D.D., Fuerch, J.H., Robinson, T.N. (2008). A randomized trial of the effects of reducing television viewing and computer use on body mass index in young children. *Archives of Pediatrics & Adolescent Medicine 162*(3), 239-245.

Francis, S., Rolls, E.T., Bowtell, R., McGlone, F., O'Doherty, J., Browning, A., Clare, S., & Smith,

E. (1999). The representation of pleasant touch in the brain and its relationship with taste and olfactory areas. *Neuroreport, 10*(3), 453-459.

Gable, S., Chang, Y., & Krull, J.L. (2007). Television watching and frequency of family meals are predictive of overweight onset and persistence in a national sample of school-aged children. *J Am Diet Assoc, 107*(1), 53-61.

Glessner, M.M., Hoover, J.H., & Halzlett, L.A. (2006). The portrayal of overweight in adolescent fiction. *Reclaiming Children and Youth, 15*(2), 116-123.

Harris, J.L., Brownell, K.D., & Bargh, J.A. (2009). The food marketing defense model: Integrating psychological research to protect youth and inform public policy. *Social Issues and Policy Review 3*(1), 211-271.

Harrison, K., & Marske, A.L. (2005). Nutritional content of foods advertised during the television programs children watch most. *Am J Public Health, 95*(9), 1568-1574.

Holmes, G. (2008). *TV, Internet and mobile usage in U.S. keeps increasing.* New York, NY: The Nielsen Company.

Huhman, M., Potter, L.D., Wong, F.L., Banspach, S.W., Duke, J.C., & Heitzler, C.D. (2005). Effects of a mass media campaign to increase physical activity among children: Year-1 results of the VERB campaign. *Pediatrics, 116*(2), e277-284.

Maher, A., Wilson, N., Signal, L., & Thomson, G. (2006). Patterns of sports sponsorship by gambling, alcohol and food companies: An Internet survey. *BMC Public Health, 6*, 95.

Martin, A. (2001). Functional neuroimaging of semantic memory. In R. Cabeza & A. Kingstone (Eds.), *Handbook of functional neuroimaging of cognition.* Cambridge, MA: The MIT Press.

Martin, A., & Chao, L. L. (2001). Semantic memory and the brain: Structure and processes. *Curr Opin Neurobiol, 11*(2), 194-201.

Martinez-Gomez, D., Tucker, J., Heelan, K.A., Welk, G.J., & Eisenmann, J.C. (2009). Associations between sedentary behavior and blood pressure in young children. *Arch Pediatr Adolesc Med, 163*(8), 724-730.

Multimedia Audiences Summary. (2003) *Statistical abstract of the United States: 2004-2005* (124th

ed., Vol. 717, Table 1121). Washington, DC: U.S. Census Bureau.

National Institute for Health and Clinical Excellence. (2009). Retrieved from www.nice.org.uk

Ogden, C.L., Carroll, M.D., & Flegal, K.M. (2008). High body mass index for age among US children and adolescents, 2003-2006. *JAMA, 299*(20), 2401-2405.

Powell, L.M., Szczypka, G., Chaloupka, F.J., & Braunschweig, C.L. (2007). Nutritional content of television food advertisements seen by children and adolescents in the United States. *Pediatrics, 120*(3), 576-583.

Rails-to-Trails Conservancy. (n.d.). TrailLink.com. Retrieved from www.traillink.com/home.aspx

Reger, B., Wootan, M.G., Booth-Butterfield, S., & Smith, H. (1998). 1% or less: A community-based nutrition campaign. *Public Health Rep, 113*(5), 410-419.

Rideout, V., Hamel, E., & Kaiser Family Foundation. (2006). *The media family: Electronic media in the lives of infants, toddlers, preschoolers and their parents.* Menlo Park: Henry J. Kaiser Family Foundation.

Simmons, W.K., Martin, A., & Barsalou, L.W. (2005). Pictures of appetizing foods activate gustatory cortices for taste and reward. *Cereb Cortex, 15*(10), 1602-1608.

Stitt, C., & Kunkel, D. (2008). Food advertising during children's television programming on broadcast and cable channels. *Health Commun, 23*(6), 573-584.

Strasburger, V.C. (2006). Children, adolescents, and advertising. *Pediatrics, 118*(6), 2563-2569.

Thompson-Schill, S.L. (2003). Neuroimaging studies of semantic memory: Inferring "how" from "where." *Neuropsychologia, 41*(3), 280-292.

Viner, R.M., & Cole, T.J. (2005). Television viewing in early childhood predicts adult body mass index. *J Pediatr, 147*(4), 429-435.

Weber, K., Story, M., & Harnack, L. (2006). Internet food marketing strategies aimed at children and adolescents: A content analysis of food and beverage brand web sites. *J Am Diet Assoc, 106*(9), 1463-1466.

INDEX

Note: The italicized *f* and *t* following page numbers refer to figures and tables, respectively.

ABOUT THE AUTHORS

Rebecca E. Lee, PhD, is the founding director of the Texas Obesity Research Center at the University of Houston. Lee is also an associate professor in the department of health and human performance at the University of Houston and holds a courtesy appointment at the University of Texas School of Public Health. She is a community health psychologist who has been principal investigator for numerous federally and privately funded research grants. Her studies have focused on interventions for populations of color, specifically interventions that incorporate social cohesion, ameliorate social injustices, and improve the quality of the neighborhood environment.

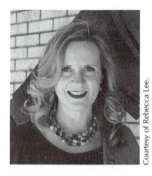
Courtesy of Rebecca Lee.

Lee serves on the editorial boards of the *International Journal of Women's Health*, the *American Journal of Health Promotion*, and *Health Psychology*. She has served as a charter member of the community-level health promotion study section of the Center for Scientific Review at the National Institutes of Health and a member and former chair of the Mayor's Wellness Council Public Policy Committee, which works to improve the health of Houstonians.

Dr. Lee is a fellow of the Society of Behavioral Medicine. She is a member of the Obesity Society and the International Society for Behavioral Nutrition and Physical Activity. She received the University of Houston College of Education Research Excellence Award in 2005 and 2008, and she has been recognized by the National Institutes of Health as a National Health Disparities Scholar. In 2009, her Saving Lives, Staying Active (SALSA) program was given the Outstanding Achievement for a Community Program Award by the Texas Council on Cardiovascular Disease and Stroke.

Kristen M. McAlexander, PhD, is a lecturer in the department of applied physiology and wellness at Southern Methodist University in Dallas, Texas. Dr. McAlexander's research interests include environmental and sociocultural influences of wellness behaviors and obesity, particularly among vulnerable populations such as women and low socioeconomic populations. McAlexander is also president and founder of Reflections Wellness, a local nonprofit organization designed to promote wellness while

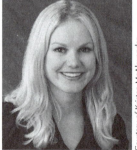
Courtesy of Kristen McAlexander.

fighting local poverty and eliminating health disparities. Her research and nonprofit organization focus on understanding and reducing health disparities and improving wellness opportunities among underserved neighborhoods.

McAlexander received a graduate research award and two graduate fellowships from the University of Houston department of health and human performance. McAlexander is an American Council on Exercise (ACE) certified personal trainer and a member of the Society for Behavioral Medicine, the American College of Sports Medicine, and the Urban Affairs Association.

Jorge A. Banda, MS, is a PhD candidate in the department of exercise science at the University of South Carolina in Columbia and a research assistant at the university's Prevention Research Center. Banda holds a master's degree in exercise science from the University of Houston. His research has focused primarily on underserved populations, including low-income-housing residents, African-American and Latina women, and low-income rural communities.

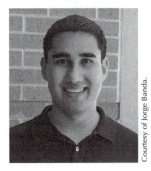

Courtesy of Jorge Banda.

Banda received a Prevention Research Center Minority Health fellowship from the Association of Schools of Public Health and the Centers for Disease Control and Prevention, and the Charles Coker Fellowship from the University of South Carolina. He was twice awarded a Norman Arnold School of Public Health fellowship. Banda also attended the Built Environment Assessment Training Institute sponsored by the U.S. Department of Agriculture, San Diego State University, and the University of Pennsylvania. He is a member of the American College of Sports Medicine and the American Public Health Association.

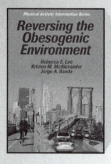
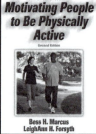
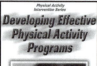

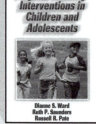